PEDIATRICS, CHILD AND ADOLESCENT HEALTH

SCHOOL, ADOLESCENCE AND HEALTH ISSUES

PEDIATRICS, CHILD AND ADOLESCENT HEALTH

JOAV MERRICK –SERIES EDITOR –

NATIONAL INSTITUTE OF CHILD HEALTH AND HUMAN DEVELOPMENT,
MINISTRY OF SOCIAL AFFAIRS, JERUSALEM, ISRAEL

Child and Adolescent Health Yearbook 2012
Joav Merrick (Editor)
2012. ISBN: 978-1-61942-788-4

Child Health and Human Development Yearbook 2011
Joav Merrick (Editor)
2012. ISBN: 978-1-61942-969-7

Tropical Pediatrics: A Public Health Concern of International Proportions
Richard R Roach, Donald E Greydanus, Dilip R Patel, Douglas N Homnick and Joav Merrick (Editors)
2012. ISBN: 8-1-61942-831-7

Developmental Issues in Chinese Adolescents
Daniel TL Shek, Rachel CF Sun and Joav Merrick (Editors)
2012. ISBN: 978-1-62081-262-4

Positive Youth Development: Theory, Research and Application
Daniel TL Shek, Rachel CF Sun and Joav Merrick (Editors)
2012. ISBN: 978-1-62081-305-8

Understanding Autism Spectrum Disorder: Current Research Aspects
Ditza A Zachor and Joav Merrick (Editors)
2012. ISBN: 978-1-62081-353-9

Positive Youth Development: A New School Curriculum to Tackle Adolescent Developmental Issues
Hing Keung Ma, Daniel TL Shek and Joav Merrick (Editors)
2012. ISBN: 978-1-62081-384-3

Transition from Pediatric to Adult Medical Care
David Wood, John G Reiss, Maria E Ferris, Linda R Edwards and Joav Merrick (Editors)
2012. ISBN: 978-1-62081-409-3

Guidelines for the Healthy Integration of the Ill Child in the Educational System: Experience from Israel
Yosefa Isenberg
2013. ISBN: 978-1-62808-350-7

Chinese Adolescent Development: Economic Disadvantages, Parents and Intrapersonal Development
Daniel TL Shek, Rachel CF Sun and Joav Merrick (Editors)
2013. ISBN: 978-1-62618-622-4

University and College Students: Health and Development Issues for the Leaders of Tomorrow
Daniel TL Shek, Rachel CF Sun and Joav Merrick (Editors)
2013. ISBN: 978-1-62618-586-9

Adolescence and Behavior Issues in a Chinese Context
Daniel TL Shek, Rachel CF Sun and Joav Merrick (Editors)
2013. ISBN: 978-1-62618-614-9

Advances in Preterm Infant Research
Jing Sun, Nicholas Buys and Joav Merrick
2013. ISBN: 978-1-62618-696-5

Internet Addiction: A Public Health Concern in Adolescence
Artemis Tsitsika, Mari Janikian, Donald E Greydanus, Hatim A Omar and Joav Merrick (Editors)
2013. ISBN: 978-1-62618-925-6

Promotion of Holistic Development of Young People in Hong Kong
Daniel TL Shek, Tak Yan Lee and Joav Merrick (Editors)
2013. ISBN: 978-1-62808-019-3

Human Developmental Research: Experience from Research in Hong Kong
Daniel TL Shek, Cecilia Ma, Yu Lu and Joav Merrick (Editors)
2013. ISBN: 978-1-62808-166-4

Chronic Disease and Disability in Childhood
Joav Merrick
2013. ISBN: 978-1-62808-865-6

Break the Cycle of Environmental Health Disparities: Maternal and Child Health Aspects
Leslie Rubin and Joav Merrick (Editors)
2013. ISBN: 978-1-62948-107-4

Environmental Health Disparities in Children: Asthma, Obesity and Food
Leslie Rubin and Joav Merrick (Editors)
2013. ISBN: 978-1-62948-122-7

Environmental Health: Home, School and Community
Leslie Rubin and Joav Merrick (Editors)
2013. ISBN: 978-1-62948-155-5

Child Health and Human Development: Social, Economic and Environmental Factors
Leslie Rubin and Joav Merrick (Editors)
2013. ISBN: 978-1-62948-166-1

Children, Violence and Bullying: International Perspectives
Joav Merrick, Isack Kandel and Hatim A Omar (Editors)
2013. ISBN: 978-1-62948-342-9

Playing with Fire: Children, Adolescents and Firesetting
Hatim A Omar, Carrie Howell Bowling and Joav Merrick (Editors)
2013. ISBN: 978-1-62948-471-6

Adolescence and Sexuality: International Perspectives
Joav Merrick, Ariel Tenenbaum and Hatim A Omar (Editors)
2014. ISBN: 978-1-62948-711-3

PEDIATRICS, CHILD AND ADOLESCENT HEALTH

SCHOOL, ADOLESCENCE AND HEALTH ISSUES

JOAV MERRICK
ARIEL TENENBAUM
AND
HATIM A. OMAR
EDITORS

New York

For permission to use material from this book please contact us:
Telephone 631-231-7269; Fax 631-231-8175
Web Site: http://www.novapublishers.com

Library of Congress Cataloging-in-Publication Data

School, adolescence, and health issues / editors, Joav Merrick, Ariel Tenenbaum, and Hatim A. Omar (medical director, Health Services, Division for Intellectual and Developmental Disabilities, Ministry of Social Affairs and Social Services, Jerusalem, Israel and others).
pages cm
Includes bibliographical references and index.
ISBN: 978-1-62948-702-1 (hardcover)
1. Teenagers--Health and hygiene. 2. Students--Health and hygiene. 3. School health services. I. Merrick, Joav, 1950- editor of compilation. II. Tenenbaum, Ariel, editor of compilation. III. Omar, Hatim A., editor of compilation.
RA777.S36 2014
613'.0433--dc23
2013045177

Published by Nova Science Publishers, Inc. † New York

CONTENTS

PREFACE

Adolescence is the critical period or rather process in human development, where the individual leaves the dependency of childhood and enters a period in which dramatic changes occur, eventually resulting in what society identifies as adulthood. It is a complex developmental time involving sociological, psychological and physiological issues that starts with puberty and ends sometime in the third decade of life with central nervous system maturation (parents would want this period to be much quicker and shorter). The goal of adolescence is to develop an autonomous adult, who is capable of functioning at intellectual, sexual, and vocational levels acceptable to society. Prevention and management of health problems in children and adolescents can prevent considerable morbidity in adults. Working with adolescents is difficult, frustrating and very rewarding at the same time. In this book, we have gathered international research to show you a picture of health issues in adolescence and during the school period of human development.

In: School, Adolescence and Health Issues
Editors: J. Merrick, A. Tenenbaum and H. A. Omar
ISBN: 978-1-62948-702-1

Chapter 1

ADOLESCENT HEALTH ISSUES

***Joav Merrick, MD, MMedSc, DMSc*[1,2,3,4,*], *Ariel Tenenbaum, MD*[1,3] *and Hatim A Omar, MD, FAAP*[4]**

[1]National Institute of Child Health and Human Development, Jerusalem, Israel
[2]Office of the Medical Director, Health Services, Division for Intellectual and Developmental Disabilities, Ministry of Social Affairs and Social Services, Jerusalem, Israel
[3]Division of Pediatrics, Hadassah Hebrew University Medical Center, Mt Scopus Campus, Jerusalem, Israel
[4]Division of Adolescent Medicine, Kentucky Children's Hospital, University of Kentucky, Lexington, Kentucky, US

Adolescence is the critical period or rather process in human development, where the individual leaves the dependency of childhood and enters a period in which dramatic changes occur, eventually resulting in what society identifies as adulthood. It is a complex developmental time involving sociological, psychological and physiological issues that starts with puberty and ends sometime in the third decade of life with central nervous system maturation (parents would want this period to be much quicker and shorter). The goal of adolescence is to develop an autonomous adult, who is capable of functioning at intellectual, sexual, and vocational levels acceptable to society.

Prevention and management of health problems in children and adolescents can prevent considerable morbidity in adults. Working with adolescents is difficult, frustrating and very rewarding at the same time. We hear all kinds of sad stories and have to live with the frustrations of not being able to wave a magic wand and change someone's life. We also see our fair share of good stories with teens doing good deeds and achieving high levels of success. It is the bad stories, however, that grab our attention, because of their sad and tragic consequences and our desire to understand why they happen.

---

[*] Correspondence: Professor Joav Merrick, MD, MMedSci, DMSc, Medical Director, Health Services, Division for Intellectual and Developmental Disabilities, Ministry of Social Affairs and Social Services, POBox 1260, IL-91012 Jerusalem, Israel. E-mail: jmerrick@zahav.net.il.

We all know that in the Western World the leading causes of mortality continue to be accidents, homicide, suicide, sexually transmitted infections, eating disorders and teen pregnancy. All are preventable yet they continue to happen. So whom should we blame? The parents for being busy and/or uneducated, the media for portraying sex, drugs and violence as a "normal" way of life, the school system for not educating our kids about real life, the health care industry that continues to deprive many of our teens access to health care, or our local and federal leaders both political and religious for giving bad examples with their continuing scandals of corruption and inappropriate sexual conduct!

It would be extremely simplistic to say that one or the other bears the blame. With the technological advances and the availability of modern communication systems including the internet, our teens are bombarded with a sea of information that is frequently inaccurate or age-inappropriate. The literature and real life experience are overall in agreement that improvement of all aspects of our societies is needed to help prevent many of our teens' problems. The parents should do their part in finding a way to spend quality time with their kids and to educate them on all aspects of life. Schools should do a better job of teaching real life skills and knowledge rather than purely academic subjects only. As a society, we should be able to provide better environment and health care for our adolescents. Our leaders should be providing good examples and so should the celebrities. If each one of us contributes, maybe we can improve our future by improving the current status of our adolescents who are our future.

About a third of youth have a chronic illness or disability and a significant number have diseases that limit daily activity. Nearly three-quarters of this group have one health condition, 21% have two, and 9% have three or more. Research suggests that 13-18% of American children and adolescents have a special health care need. Approximately 90% of children with severe illness reach age 20 years in developed countries, and the impact of chronic illness on the lives of these children and adolescents is considerable.

In this book we have brought together papers that discuss various aspects of adolescent health, behaviors, parenting and educating adolescents from different countries and different cultures.

SECTION ONE: SCHOOL HEALTH ISSUES

In: School, Adolescence and Health Issues
Editors: J. Merrick, A. Tenenbaum and H. A. Omar
ISBN: 978-1-62948-702-1

Chapter 2

ALLERGIES AMONG ELEMENTARY SCHOOL CHILDREN: INTEGRATION OF DAILY ENVIRONMENTAL AND SCHOOL HEALTH SURVEILLANCE SYSTEMS

Wasantha P Jayawardene, MD*[*,1], Ahmed H Youssef Agha, PhD[2] and David K Lohrmann, PhD[1]

[1]Department of Applied Health Science
[2]Department of Epidemiology and Biostatistics,
School of Public Health Bloomington, Indiana University, Indiana,
United States of America

ABSTRACT

In this chapter we try to determine if a relationship exists between occurrence of allergies among elementary school children and daily upper-air observations (temperature, relative humidity, dew point, mixing ratio) and to derive a mathematical model that predicts allergies. Using an ecological study design, school health records of 168,825 students in elementary schools enrolled in "Health eTools for Schools" within 49 Pennsylvania counties were analyzed. Data representing asthma exacerbations were originally recorded by school nurses as the type of treatment given to a student during a clinic visit on a particular day. Daily upper-air measurements from ground level to the 850mb pressure level, covering a radius of 800 kilometers around Pittsburg, PA, were obtained. Wilcoxon Two-Sample test was used to identify associations. A Generalized Estimating Equation model was used to predict the occurrence of more than 13 cases, the daily mean for 2008-2010. Results showed that the surveillance of allergies among school children in Pennsylvania is increased over last three years. The primary occurrence of allergies among school children was in August-September, followed by December and April, while the lowest in January and May. Annual averages of upper-air observations were

[*] Correspondence: Wasantha P Jayawardene, MD, Doctoral Candidate and Associate Instructor, Department of Applied Health Science, Room 116, School of Public Health Bloomington, Indiana University, 1025 E 7th Street, Bloomington, IN 47405, United States. E-mail: wajayawa@indiana.edu.

significantly different between seasons (p<0.02). Upper-air temperature, dew point, and mixing ratio above their three-year mean values were significantly associated with occurrence of allergies (p<0.011). In conclusion, monitoring of upper-air observation data over time can be a reliable means for predicting outbreaks of allergies among elementary school children. Such predictions could help parents and school nurses implement effective precautionary measures.

INTRODUCTION

Hay fever, respiratory allergies, food allergies, and skin allergies are the main types of allergies among children in the United States. Percent of children with diagnosed hay fever in the past 12 months is 9.5% (7.1 million), while 11.5% (3.4 million) of children reported with respiratory allergies. In addition, 4.6% (9.4 million) of children in the US had food allergies in the past 12 months, while 12.6% of children reported with skin allergies (1).Seasonal allergies are fairly common in children older than age of five year. According to the American Academy of Allergy, Asthma, and Immunology, about 10-15% of school-age children have seasonal allergies (2). According to CDC, about 10% of children under 17 years had suffered from hay fever, 12% from respiratory allergies, 5% from food allergies, and 13% from skin allergies in the past 12 months (3). There is some evidence that more than 10% of children were sensitized to pollen and a high proportion of the children sensitized only to pollen were also sensitized to other inhalant allergens later. Technically, an allergen is a non-parasitic antigen capable of stimulating a type-1 hypersensitivity reaction in atopic individuals (4). The most common allergens are: pollen, dust, food, insect stings, animal dander, mold, medications, and latex. Most humans mount significant Immunoglobulin E (IgE) responses only as a defense against parasitic infections. However, some individuals mount an IgE response against common environmental antigens (4).

Seasonality of allergies (5, 6) and their association with asthma (7) are well-known phenomena. Atopic eczema and allergic rhinitis were found to be higher in period September–May. Some evidence support that non-summer warmth and urban air pollution (8), probably mediated through exposure to common allergens such as dust mites, are possible risk factors for allergies in school-aged children (9). The highest frequencies of IgE reactivity to food were found in the group of children sensitized to several types of pollen (10).

Seasonal allergy symptoms are commonly experienced due to pollen in summer, fall, or spring, when certain trees or grasses pollinate. The season of pollination depends on the type of tree or grass. As an example, grasses such as Bermuda, timothy and orchard pollinate in the summer, while some trees such as oak, elm, and maple pollinate in the spring. Grass allergy is generally linked to hay fever because their symptoms and causes are somehow similar to each other. Symptoms include rhinitis, which causes sneezing, and a runny nose, as well as allergic conjunctivitis, which includes watering and itchy eyes (2). Also, depending on the season, the symptoms may be more severe. The immune system has strong influence on seasonal allergies, since it reacts differently to diverse allergens like pollen. Meteorological factors are very important for the occurrence of pollen grains in the air. Dry and hot weather speeds up maturation and the loosening of pollen grains from anthers, and the concentration of pollen grains is considerably higher than in cold and wet weather (11). It is found that the temperature has a positive correlation with pollen count, while relative humidity has an inverse correlation with the pollen count in the atmosphere. The total daily rainfall is also has a negative correlation (11). Wind and thunderstorms are also accelerating the process of pollen release, especially in spring and summer months (12).

The current study investigated was undertaken to determine if a relationship exists between occurrence of allergies among school children, based on school health services records, and routine upper-air variables, such as mixing ratio, relative humidity, temperature, and dew point. Mixing ratio is the mass of water vapor per unit mass of dry air, while relative humidity is the partial pressure of water vapor in air, given as a percentage of the saturated vapor pressure under the same conditions. Air temperature at which condensation first begins is the dew point, another measure of humidity. Although temperature and relative humidity at ground surface level have been extensively considered in asthma studies, neither dew point nor mixing ratio have been linked with asthma or used for prediction of asthma outbreaks. The concept of relative humidity is complex. The amount of humidity is relative to the temperature available to do the work of evaporation, and can fluctuate even if no change occurs in the actual amount of water vapor per unit mass of dry air (mixing ratio). Therefore, dew point and mixing ratio provide the best assessments of humidity as it relates to asthma exacerbations.

The atmospheric variables examined in this study are upper-air observations. Upper air observations constitute measurements of atmospheric conditions at higher altitudes, as distinct from surface weather observations, which are evaluations of the state of the atmosphere as observed at a point on the earth's surface and a set of instruments sent by a free-flight balloon (radiosonde), measures atmospheric variables from the surface to aheightof6 to30 km (troposphere and stratosphere), and transmits the data to aground receiving system. Radiosondes typically measure temperature, dew point, mixing ratio, relative humidity, and sometimes, pressure and wind speed/direction (13). The US National Weather Service's Upper-Air Observation Program monitors the operation of92radiosondestations in North America and the Pacific islands. Observations are updated twice daily. Temperature normally decreases throughout the troposphere as altitude increases. This phenomenon is called the lapse rate which, on average, occurs in the troposphere at a rate of 3.6°F per 1,000 ft. This means that a strong, consistent correlation exists between upper-air temperatures and ground temperatures. None of these daily upper-air observation parameters described above has been utilized in asthma research to date, either to detect associations or for prediction of asthma outbreaks.

School health records have been utilized for asthma-tracking because they are readily accessible through the existing school data collection and storage infrastructure (14). In many Pennsylvania schools student health records are compiled through a web-based software application portal called "Health eTools for Schools" (hereafter referred to as "eTools") that was funded by the Highmark Foundation through its Healthy High Five Initiative (15) and developed by InnerLink, Inc, a private, for-profit company.. With the utilitarian purpose of providing data for state and local health planning, eTools is provided free of charge to local public, private and parochial schools. Implemented in approximately 1,100 schools in 49 Pennsylvania counties located in or near the Pittsburgh area, eTools is used by school nurses to routinely collect student health record data. The School Health Services section of eTools allows nurses to efficiently enter and download student health data using a hand-held electronic device, and via computerized programming, compile and submit required annual reports to the Pennsylvania State Health Department. Our study involved analysis of existing de-identified student health record information pertaining to asthma exacerbations that was routinely collected and aggregated in the eTools data management system by school nurses.

OUR STUDY

Ecological study design was adopted in order to understand the relationship between daily occurrence of asthma in a "whole population" of elementary school students and daily measurements of upper-air observation parameters (16). In the ecological design, which investigates group-level variables, a geographical region can be analyzed in a cross-sectional manner (once or repetitively) to investigate the variation in a health-related variable (e.g., mean blood pressure, hospitalizations for asthma, and homicide rates) and its associations with regional characteristics (e.g., salt intake, air pollution, handgun laws, and drug policies) (16).

Two categories of group-level variables are found in epidemiological study designs. The first is aggregate variables; summary measures of individual characteristics (e.g., per capita income). These variables demonstrate a distinction between individual-level and group-level characteristics, because the group-level measure is inferior to (a weaker measure than) the individual-level measure. The second is integral variables; group-level variables that are not summary measures of individual-level variables (e.g., weather, air pollution, and laws). These variables do not have corresponding individual-level values and can only be investigated at the group-level.

Since upper-air variables in the current study are integral variables, ecological study design is the most appropriate analytic approach.

An ecological design also has the advantageous ability to control for individual-level variability while at the same time addressing influences at the regional-level. In addition, this study design enables researchers to include all the students of the enrolled elementary schools in the study sample, contrary to a study design in which each student with an allergic condition serves as his/her own control and excludes other students (16). Moreover, extracting daily upper-air data from existing environmental databases and retrieving computerized daily health data from existing repositories, such as eTools, is inherently cost-effective in that it requires a very low level of effort.

Study population

School districts located in 49 of the 67 counties in Pennsylvania participated in eTools. From 2008 to 2010, enrolled school districts received eTools services for 168,825 elementary school students. These students constituted the study population. All eTools services for participating school districts were subsidized by the founders of eTools (Highmark Foundation) and covered costs of utilizing eTools through a three-year period. School districts that opted into eTools had to meet five requirements in order to receive a fully paid subscription service: 1) Make a three year commitment to use the portal, 2) Increase the amount of instructional time spent on nutrition education to 75 minutes per marking period,

3) Provide increased opportunities for physical education and physical activity through age appropriate instruction, 4) Participate in in-service training and professional development offerings that enhance use of the portal, 5) Participate in an annual evaluation of eTools effectiveness. Pennsylvania schools that met participation criteria were eligible to be covered under the subsidy program during the three-year period and were considered for participation on a first-come, first-served basis.

Therefore, all students attending the 1,100 schools in participating school districts were represented by eTools. At the individual level, the sole participation eligibility requirement was to be a student with a health record in an elementary school that utilized eTools. Student records from these schools were excluded if they contained incomplete or inaccurately entered health record data.

In addition, no race-, ethnicity-, or income-based bias existed in the enrollment of schools districts, schools, or students in eTools. All of the above factors are important in respect to generalizability of study results to elementary school students at the state level or beyond the state level (16).

Data collection

Within the 49 Pennsylvania counties, 168,825records of elementary school students were identified for this study. Data on asthma were originally noted in records maintained by school nurses as the type of treatment given to a student on a particular day. Treatment options for school health nurses were based on the prescribed medication provided for the student. For purposes of this study, having allergy was defined as "any case managed with antihistamines". In fact, school nurses recorded the trade name of all the medications administered, which were then later categorized into functional groups (i.e., anti-asthmatics, analgesics, etc.). It was assumed that the treatment option noted by a school nurse correctly represented the disease.

Data analyzed for this study were provided to the authors by InnerLink, Inc. which had custorial responsibility under a common Statement of Understanding and Service Level Agreement with all participating school systems. Data pertaining to total use of antiasthmatic medications at the school level was unavailable. Likewise, demographic characteristics of students in each school or school district were not included in the eTools database and, therefore, were unobtainable.

The school year in Pennsylvania usually begins in August, ends in June and typically includes an extended winter break. Therefore, surveillance data were commonly unavailable for the last three weeks of June, all of July, the first three weeks of August, and the second half of December every year.

According to Pennsylvania State regulations, each school entity (e.g., school district) must have a written policy to allow for the possession and self-administration by school-age children of an asthma inhaler and the prescribed medication to be administered thereby in a school setting (17). The policy under this section shall require a child of school age that desires to possess and self-administer an asthma inhaler in a school setting to demonstrate the capability for self-administration and for responsible behavior in the use of an asthma inhaler. The physician, certified registered nurse practitioner or physician assistant shall state whether the child is qualified and able to self-administer the medication. A written request is also required from the parent or guardian to the effect that the school entity complies with the order of the physician, certified registered nurse practitioner or physician assistant (17).

Because of these regulations, which rely on developmentally-appropriate restrictions on self-administration of medications for allergies, while allowed on an individual basis at any age, is less likely to occur among elementary school students. The number of visits by middle school and high school students to school health nurse's office, therefore, may not accurately represent the number of allergy occurrences. Hence, only data from elementary school students' records were included in this study.

All US schools districts, including those in Pennsylvania, must collect and maintain all student records, including health records, in accordance with provisions of the federal Family Educational Rights and Privacy Act (FERPA).

Regardless of whether a school is in a contractual arrangement with Innerlink, school nurses must maintain proper records safeguards; therefore, participation in eTools created no added burden for nurses in participating schools. FERPA regulations also give states the flexibility to share data for the purpose of ensuring that taxpayer funds are invested wisely in programs as long as students' personal information is properly safeguarded (18).

This study involved analysis of existing de-identified student health record information pertaining to asthma exacerbations that was routinely collected and aggregated in the eTools data management system by school nurses who followed all FERPA safeguards. A common contract with InnerLink holds school districts responsible for maintaining the privacy, confidentiality and integrity of all data, systems and intellectual property related to eTools. InnerLink requirements affirmed that all school districts adhere to the FERPA regulations of 1974.

Upper-air observation data were utilized for this study, for three reasons: 1) they are closely correlated with surface weather observations; 2) upper-air observations are following the same protocol as common for all locations in Pennsylvania, so a single value can be used for the entire state; 3) no study has tested the association and usefulness of upper-air observations in allergy research. The upper-air data used in this study were downloaded from the Wyoming University web site (13).

Measurements were obtained from the ground level to1500 meters level (which is equivalent to 850 mb pressure). These upper-air observation values cover an area with a radius of about 800 kilometers, around Pittsburg, PA (Figure 1).

As the coverage area includes the whole state of Pennsylvania, the geographical distribution of schools within the state did not affect study results. For each day of the three years (2008-2010) the measured values at time12Z were obtained for analysis. The Z-time is the basis for synoptic meteorology, which requires collection of all measurements at the same time every day and, thereby, produces a snapshot of the state of the atmosphere worldwide. The12Ztimein the United States is 6 a.m. in January (Eastern Standard Time) and 7a.m. in July (Eastern Daylight Time).

This particular time was selected, because7 a.m. is closer to the usual time when students travel to school and are exposed to outdoor climatic factors. Due to this, any difference between the outside air temperature and the air temperature in the school is irrelevant. The variation of upper-air measurement values over the day is very small; the range of upper-air temperature over a day is less than 5^0 F (13).

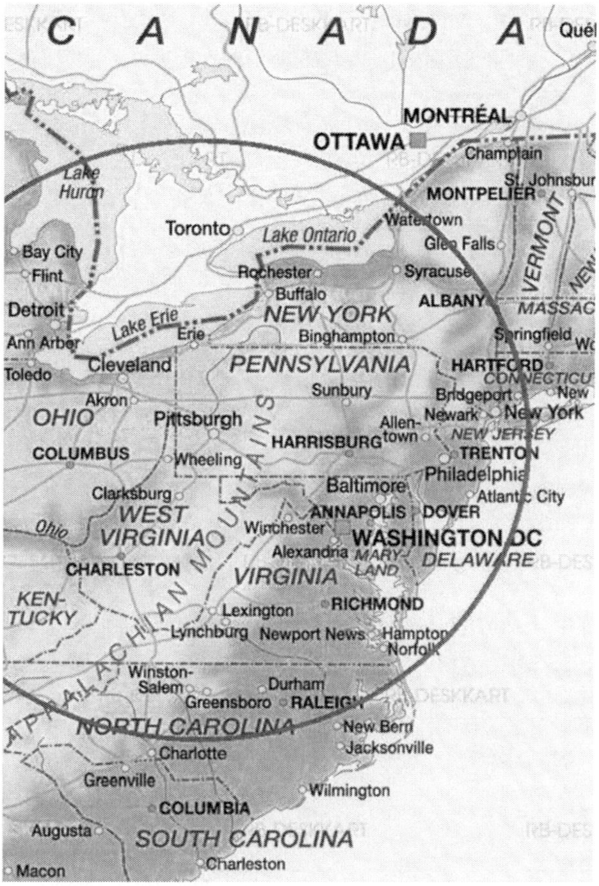

Figure 1. Map of Pennsylvania and Surrounding States Depicting Coverage Area of Upper-Air Observation Data, which is Equal to a Radius of 800 km Around Pittsburgh.

Analysis

Descriptive statistics were used to summarize the mean changes of allergy cases throughout years. Two ratios were created: 1) daily mean allergy cases to annual average of allergy cases; 2) daily mean of allergy cases to number of schools enrolled. The first ratio was employed to study relationships between upper-air observation factors and allergies, and the second ratio was used to study the pattern of allergy occurrences over years. A nonparametric test, the Wilcoxon Two-Sample test, was used to compare means of first ratio that correspond to low and high groups of upper-air observations (with cutoff at three year median). Chi Square test was used to identify associations between the relative humidity (with cutoff at relative humidity=50%) and occurrence of allergies.

Generalized Estimating Equation (GEE) model was used to predict the probability of occurrence of cases greater than or equal to 13 (a cutoff value equal to the 2008-2010 mean). The repeated subject (cluster) in the model is the "matched date," for example, March 8th in 2007, 2008, 2009, and in 2010 is a subject. GEE needs at least 100 clusters to study5-12exploratoryvariables, however, a great deal of confidence is assured with 200 clusters, (19, 20) the circumstance in in the current study. "Logit" link function on binary distribution was used on a binary dependent variable. "P" represents DailyAllergyCases≥13 and "1-P" represents Daily Allergy Cases<13. The independent variables were the upper-air observation variables.

The study was approved by the Indiana University Bloomington Institutional Review Board, Bloomington, Indiana, United States.

FINDINGS

Offices of school health nurses in Pennsylvania had 259,951 visits of elementary school students for various health problems during the three year period, 2008-2010 (Table 1). This was equal to 40.9% of total student visits (preK-12) for the period. The treatment option in more than 60% of these occasions was either analgesics (30.7%) or Attention Deficit Hyperactivity Disorder drugs (30.0%). Antihistamines were given in 1.61% of occasions, which reflected the occurrence of this disease or disease exacerbations among students of all grades.

Table 1. Student Visits to Offices of School Nurses for Various Types of Treatments in Pennsylvania, preK-12 and preK-5, during 2008-2010, and Daily Means for the Period

Disease	No. of Visits by preK-12	No. of Visits by preK-5	% of Visits by preK-5	Daily Mean preK-5	Daily Median preK-5	Daily St Dev preK-5
ADHDs	190,992	110,833	58.00%	194	188	99
Analgesics	195,449	38,079	19.50%	67	66	36
Anti-asthmatics	39,185	27,123	69.20%	48	45	27
Anti-diabetics	65,361	26,440	40.50%	46	45	25
Gastrointestinals	60,318	22,601	37.50%	40	40	21
Antibiotics	27,070	15,585	57.60%	27	25	21
Other Psychotropics	22,135	9,121	41.20%	16	16	9
Antihistamines	8,546	4,185	49.00%	7	6	6
Anticonvulsants	8,838	3,461	39.20%	6	6	3
Anti-inflammatories	18,189	2,523	13.90%	4	3	4
Total	636,083	259,951	40.9%			

A gradual increase of allergy cases was observed from 2008 to 2010, both in elementary schools and in schools with higher grades (Table 2). This is partially explained by the increase in the number of schools participating in the allergy surveillance system. The total number of schools (elementary, middle, and high) increased from 2008 to 2009, with a slight decrease from 2009 to 2010.

Table 2. Visits to School Health Nurses Due to Allergy as Reported by School Heath Nurses in Pennsylvania, 2007-2010

Year	Number of Schools	Avg. of Allergy Daily Visits (preK-5)	Ratio of [Daily Cases/Schools] for the Year
2008	471	4 (SD=3)	0.85
2009	675	7 (SD=5)	1.04
2010	621	11 (SD=8)	1.77

However, a boost from 0.85 to 1.77 (208% increase) in the ratio of daily average of allergy cases to number of schools (preK-5) partially explained the real increase in allergy prevalence among school children, because that particular increase is not influenced by an increase in the number of schools participating in the allergy surveillance system. It may, however, be influenced by increased reporting of school nurses, since any surveillance system takes a few years to reach the full functional capacity. Geographical differences in new school enrolment may also have influenced this 208% increase. Differences between daily means of allergy cases reported from elementary schools in each year (2008, 2009, and 2010) were statistically significant ($p<0.001$; Kruskal-Wallis test). This statistical significance is true for both the daily mean, and the ratio of daily cases to annual average ($p<0.004$).

Use of antihistamines among school children as reported by school health nurses has an almost identical pattern in each year during 2008-2010 (Figure 2). Peak of antihistamine use lies in period from late August to early September, although there are noticeable increases in December (early winter) and in April (early spring) too. The lowest use of antihistamine use is reported in January and in May (Figure 2).

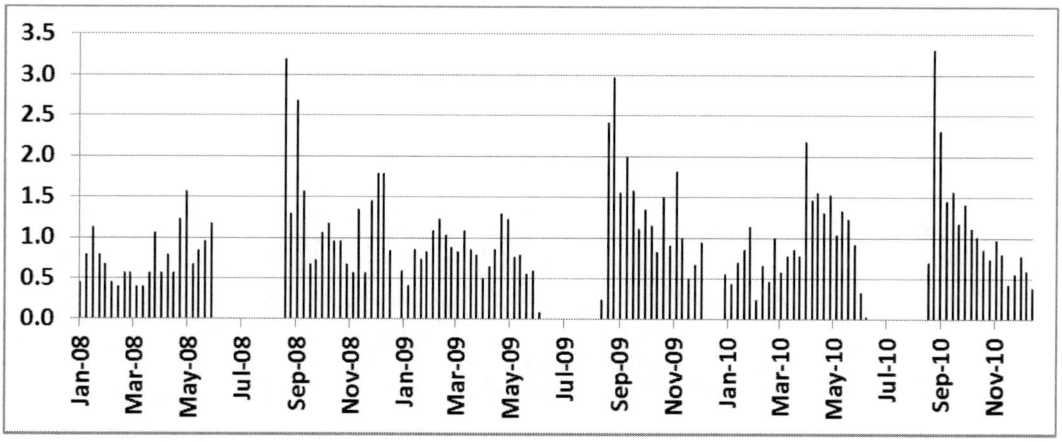

*No data available for the period between 25th and 34th week of the year due to summer vacation; No data available for the last (52nd) week of the year due to winter break.

Figure 2. Antihistamine Use among preK-5 Students (Ratio of Weekly Mean to Annual Mean), 2008-2010*.

It should be considered that the last three weeks of June, whole month of July, and first three weeks of August have no surveillance due to summer vacation as well as the second half of December has no reporting due to winter break. Differences between daily means of allergy cases reported from elementary schools in each season were statistically significant (p<0.001) according to Kruskal-Wallis test. This significance is not only true for daily mean, but also true for the ratio of daily cases to annual average as well (p<0.001). As winter has the lowest number of cases, it was considered the baseline for number of allergy cases in odds ratio estimates. The summer season compared to winter, had 17 times higher tendency of exceeding daily mean of allergy cases (7 cases), which was followed by fall (2.6 times higher), and spring (2.1 times higher). In other words, 68% of days in summer exceeded daily mean of allergy cases for three years, followed by fall (38%), and spring (35%).

Upper-air temperature peaks in July (hot) and has its minimum in January (cold). Non of the annual means of four upper-air observations showed difference between years according to Kruskal-Wallis test. There were significant differences between temperature means for each season (p<0.001), with the highest in summer, followed by spring, and then fall (Figure 3). Similarly, upper-air dew point peaks in July (wet) and reaches its minimum in January (dry). Significant differences existed between seasons (p<0.001), with the highest in summer, followed by spring, and then fall (Figure 4). Significant differences between mixing ratio means for each season were also statistically significant (p<0.001), with the highest in summer, followed by spring, and fall. Variation in upper-air relative humidity is complex and it's difficult to identify a specific pattern (Figure 5). Differences between relative humidity means for each season were statistically significant (p<0.02), with the highest in summer, followed by winter, and then fall. The lowest relative humidity was recorded in spring.

Wilcoxon two-sample test was used to determine the significance of association between allergy cases reported from elementary schools during three years (2008-2010) and each upper-air observation indicator (Table 3). The ratio of daily allergy cases to annual average was utilized for analysis instead of using the absolute number of daily allergy cases to minimize the effect of increase in allergy reporting over three years. The ratio of allergy occurrence has statistically significant associations with all four upper-air observation indicators.

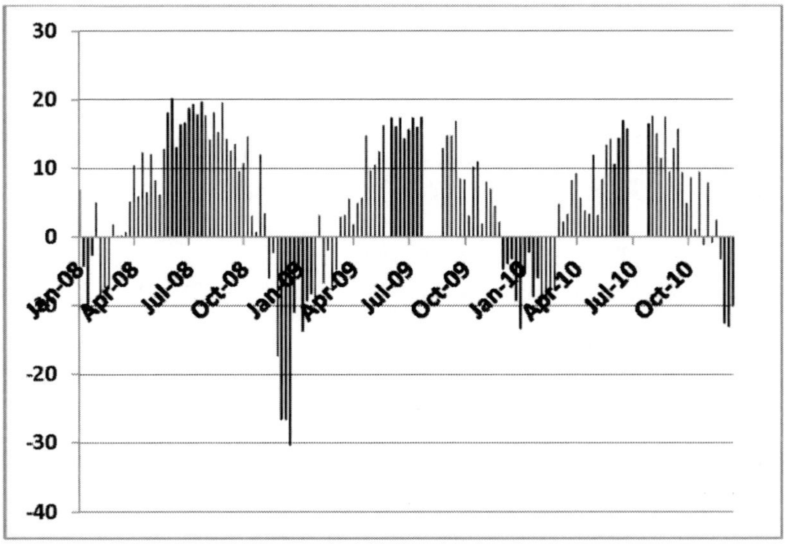

Figure 3. Fluctuation of Weekly Mean of Upper-Air Temperature (Celsius), 2008-2010.

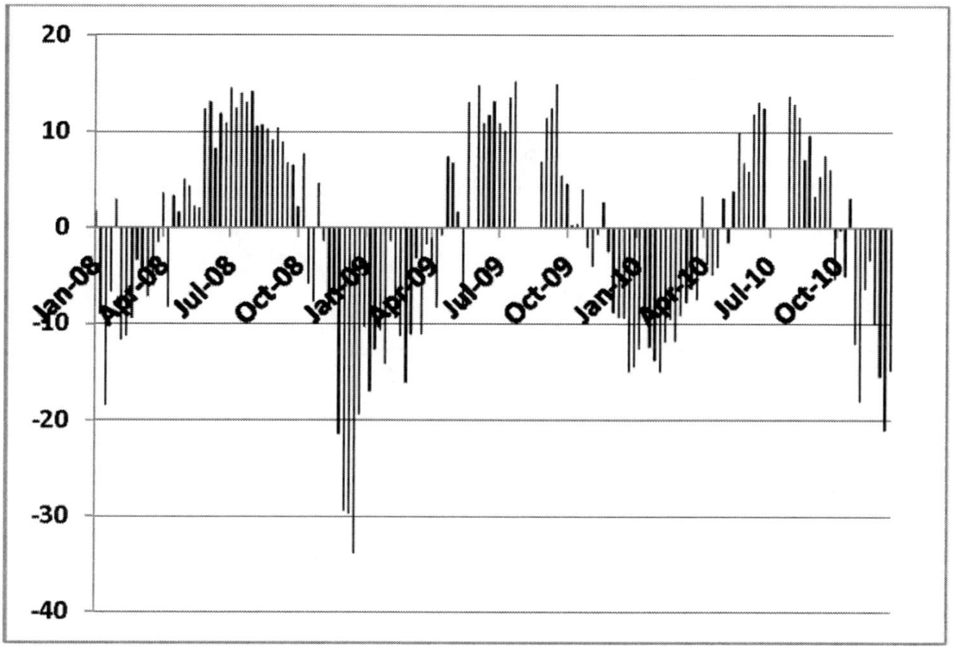

Figure 4. Fluctuation of Weekly Mean of Upper-Air Dew Point (Celsius), 2008-2010.

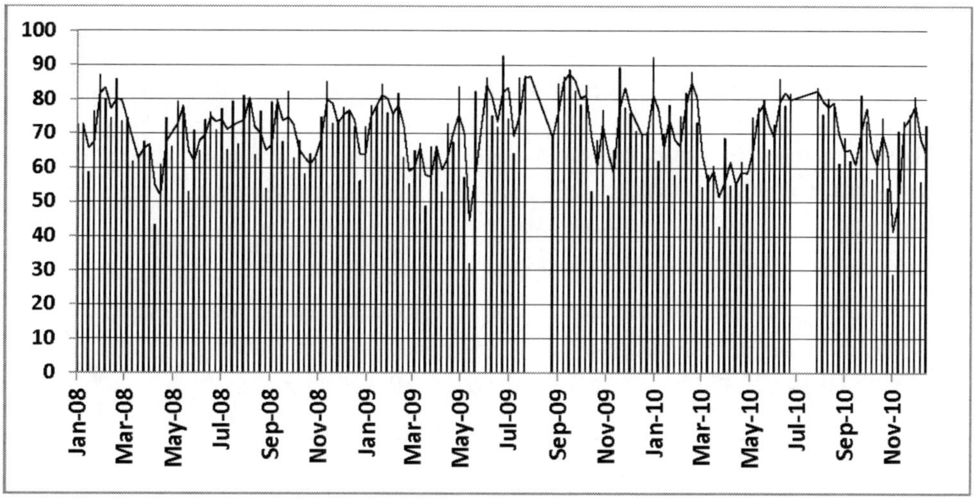

Figure 5. Fluctuation of Weekly Mean of Relative Humidity (Percent), 2008-2010.

Cut off points for dew point, temperature, and mixing ratio were considered as the median values (for three year period) of each variable: -3.42, 4.36, and 2.92 respectively. When the upper-air dew point was higher than its median value, the occurrence of allergy cases was higher and this difference was statistically significant ($p<0.0001$).

Similarly, higher number of cases reported with a higher value of upper-air mixing ratio ($p<0.0001$). Finally, when the upper-air temperature was higher than its median value, a higher number of allergy cases were reported ($p<0.0006$).

The cut off for relative humidity (50%) was obtained using guidelines from Mayo Clinic and American College of Allergy, Asthma, and Immunology (ACAAI) (21, 22). The Chi-Square test revealed that relative humidity had no significant association with occurrence of allergy cases. Lastly, the Chi Square test revealed that season, mixing ratio, and interaction of temperature with relative humidity are important in determining whether or not the number of allergy cases is greater than the daily mean of allergy cases for the particular year.

Table 3. Comparing Means of Allergy Cases Ratio[1] by Low/High Classes of Upper-air Observations, 2008-2010

Dew Point[§] (^{0}C)	N	Mean Of Ratio[Ψ]	SD	Wilcoxon Test
DWPT > -3.42	296	1.125	0.849	Pr< 0.0001
DWPT <= -3.42	272	0.887	0.675	
Mix Ratio[§] (g/kg)				
MIXR >4.36	236	1.181	0.902	Pr< 0.0001
MIXR<=4.36	332	0.886	0.647	
Temperature[§] (^{0}C)				
Temp >2.92	305	1.130	0.851	Pr< 0.0006
Temp<=2.92	263	0.878	0.666	

[Ψ] Allergy Cases Ratio = Daily Cases / Annual Average.
[§]The cutoff values are three-year median values for dew point, mixing ratio, and temperature.

Finally, using the GEE model, the following equation was adopted for determining the probability of having ≥13 cases (three year mean + one standard deviation) on a day:

$$y = a_0 + a_1x_1 + a_2x_2 + a_3x_3 + a_4 (x_4*x_2)$$

$$\log \frac{P}{1-P} = -4.3212 - 0.2685 (T) - 2.4288 (MR) - 0.1012 (RH) - 0.074 (DP * MR)$$

log P/(1-P) = Logarithm of odds ratio for the [mean + one standard deviation] cases (=13 cases) on a day

P = Probability of having ≥13 allergy cases on a particular day
1 – P = Probability of having allergies on that day
T = Upper-air temperature ^{0}C (in Celsius)
MR = Upper-air actual mixing ratio g/kg (in grams per kilogram)
RH = Relative humidity % (in percent)
DP = Upper-air dew point temperature ^{0}C (in Celsius)

As an example, if the upper-air temperature, upper-air mixing ratio, upper-air relative humidity, and upper-air dew point temperature are 12^{0}C, 5 g/kg, 55%, and 5^{0}C respectively on a particular day, the probability (P) of having more than 13 cases of allergies within the surveillance system on that day is 64%.

Discussion

The surveillance of allergy among school children in Pennsylvania has improved during last four years in both aspects: the school enrollment in the surveillance system and the disease reporting by school health nurses, a proven, reliable data source (23). The increased exposure to allergens and changes in other socioeconomic and sociodemographic factors among school children may be the main reasons for increase in allergies in Pennsylvania. The finding of the current study that peaks (main outbreaks) of allergy occurrence were reported in August-September and in April was compatible with above evidence from empirical studies. However, having the highest prevalence in summer months may be associated with characteristics of pollen that cause allergic symptoms (2).

Annual averages of upper-air observations (temperature, relative humidity, dew point, mixing ratio) did not differ between years. As explained previously, a higher temperature (greater than three year median) is associated with occurrence of more allergies among Pennsylvania school children. However, this study considered only the upper-air temperature, not the surface level ambient temperature. Similarly, a higher upper-air dew point was found to be related to the occurrence of more allergies. In addition, a higher upper-air mixing ratio was associated with occurrence of more allergies. The review of literature found no record of these latter two associations. It's important that all three associations were considered in isolation during the analysis, rather than assessing their interaction with each other or with any other variable, such as relative humidity, air pollution, or pollen. The upper-air relative humidity showed no association with occurrence of allergies at its median value cut off, although the upper-air relative humidity ≥50% was significantly associated with allergies. As discussed previously, the concept of relative humidity is complex, because relative humidity is relative to the amount of energy (measured by temperature) available to do the work of evaporation, and it can be changed without having any change in the actual amount of water vapor in the air (absolute humidity). Therefore, dew point and actual mixing ratio in conjunction with temperature provide a better assessment of humidity, which is more relevant to allergies.

Put another way, the routinely measured and publicly available upper-air indicators provide a good estimate and a reliable tool for forecasting allergy burden on the school health system today or on a future day. This output of analysis with GEE is based on a three-year mean of allergies (13 cases) and does not restrict the utilization of the above equation beyond interpolation. Therefore, the extrapolation for forecasting is also realistic given the current analysis, based on the average of allergies for the 2008-2010 period.

Apart from decreased accuracy that results from using group averages and ignoring individual level variations, a risk of occurring "ecological fallacy" also exists; the erroneous interpretation that specific asthmatic children in the group share the characteristics of the study sample. In prediction of incidence, it is inappropriate to infer that a specific asthmatic child has an X% probability of experiencing an asthma exacerbation on a particular day. However, it is possible to interpret that there is an X% probability of more than N number of asthma exacerbation occurrences in the study sample on a particular day (16). In addition, there is a possibility that other asthma triggers, such as pollen, air pollution, and respiratory infections, may confound the relationship between upper-air variables and asthma exacerbations.

Asthma surveillance in schools is not being conducted during winter break and summer vacations, as well as during weekends and school holidays. The relatively less data available for the summer season due to school vacation may somewhat distort the relationships caused by unequal representativeness across seasons.

In addition, it is difficult to exclude the possibility that some students who experience worsening of symptoms at night or early in the morning did not attend the school so their asthma exacerbations are not included in school health records. It was also impossible to estimate the number of students with respiratory symptoms who did not receive medications in school or who received medication that was not administered by a nurse as some elementary school students may have taken asthma medications without informing the school nurse. Therefore, we cannot exclude the possibility that use of antiasthmatic medications as recorded by school nurse somewhat under-represented the occurrence of asthmatic symptoms at school. Unavailability of antiasthmatic medications usage data at school level as well as absence of data on demographic characteristics (e.g., ethnicity, income) of students in each school or school district were also limitations.

The number of schools using eTools during 2007 was relatively low and, therefore, student data from that year were not included in some of the analyses. The number of schools using eTools changed each year with some schools dropping off and others joining, causing fluctuations in the total number of available student data records. Additionally, each year some students were leaving their school or school district. Nevertheless, the total number of student data strings provided for anyone year was sufficiently robust, as was the number of data strings available for multi-year comparisons, to generate reliable results.

Both respiratory and skin allergies may have an association with upper-air variables and both can also be caused by food allergies. Unfortunately, no mechanism exists for distinguishing respiratory and skin allergies from food allergies, because school nurses did not specify the type of allergy associated with treatments they provided. Therefore, we cannot exclude the possibility that a distortion of the relationship between upper-air indicators and respiratory and skin allergies occurred due to the inclusion of food allergies in the analysis. Most probably, a causal relationship between upper-air observations and occurrence of food allergy symptoms does not exist; however, the seasonality of some food allergies is an observed phenomenon possibly caused by seasonal fluctuations in sunlight, and perhaps vitamin D (24).

Finally, as we cannot exclude the confounding effect of pollen on relationship between climatic factors and allergies, another study will be conducted utilizing the same data sources to evaluate the combined effect of pollen in combination with climatic factors on allergies.

CONCLUSION

The surveillance of allergies among school children in Pennsylvania increased over three years in two aspects: school enrollment in surveillance system and the allergy reporting by school health nurses, a proven reliable source. The primary occurrence of allergies among elementary school children was in August-September, followed by April, although the highest overall prevalence was reported in summer, followed by fall. The lowest incident of allergies was reported in winter. Annual averages of upper-air observations (temperature, relative humidity, dew point, mixing ratio) were significantly different between seasons. Upper-air temperature, dew point, and mixing ratio above their three-year mean values were significantly associated with occurrence of allergies, although upper-air relative humidity ≥50% was not.

Monitoring of upper-air observation data (temperature, dew point, and actual mixing ratio) over time can serve as a reliable means for predicting increased occurrence of allergies among elementary school children. The new mathematical model derived from statistical integration of routine environmental observations and school health records may be used to scrutinize the complexity of allergic diseases as a dynamic outcome determined by multiple environmental parameters. It's also possible to assess the risk for future allergy outbreaks based on fluctuation analysis of a long time series of atmospheric function.

Predicting of allergy outbreaks is important for children diagnosed as having allergies and their household members can take more preventive measures to avoid allergic conditions, regardless of the severity of allergic condition. In addition, being informed of a possible allergy outbreak on a particular day or week, teachers will be able to pay more attention on early identification of allergic reactions among children in the classroom. Being informed of a possible allergy outbreak, doctors and nurses in emergency room or in the family practice can take extra preparations and utilize resources more efficiently to serve an increased number of allergy patients. With accurate prediction, the school health system can also play a major role by effectively reallocating both human and physical resources as well as by alarming teachers and children with allergies to take extra precautions and identify allergic reactions very early. Mass media and local media can also play an important role in all of these aspects. Results of the current study can be used to inform similar programming at the national level and in other states. Monitoring of upper-air observation data over time can serve as a reliable means for predicting outbreaks of allergies among elementary school children for taking more effective precautionary measures.

Acknowledgments

Authors thank InnerLink Inc for developing eTools and also Highmark Foundation of Pittsburgh, Pennsylvania for implementing Highmark Healthy High 5 Initiative. The authors report no conflicts of interest in relation to the current study.

References

[1] Centers for Disease Control and Prevention. Fast Stats: Allergies and hay fever. URL: http://www.cdc.gov/nchs/fastats/allergies.htm.

[2] American Academy of Allergy, Asthma, and Immunology. Allergies. URL: http://www.aaaai.org/conditions-and-treatments/allergies.aspx.

[3] United States Department of Health and Human Services. Summary Health Statistics for U.S. Children: National Health Interview Survey, 2010. Hyattsville, MD: Centers Disease Control Prevention, National Center Health Statistics, PHS-2012-1578,250, 2011.

[4] Goldsby RA, et al. Immunology, 5 ed. New York: WH Freeman, 2000.

[5] Ricard N, Sauriol L, Christian S. Burden of care and quality of life amongst parents of children with seasonal allergies. J Allergy Clin Immunol 1999;103(1):S72-S.

[6] Moller C, Elsayed S. Seasonal variation of the conjunctival provocation test: Total and specific IGE in children with birch pollen allergy. Int Arch Allergy Appl Immunol 1990;92(3):306-8.

[7] Kurt E, Metintas S, Basyigit I, Bulut I, Coskun E, Dabak S, et al. Prevalence and risk factors of allergies in Turkey: Results of a multi-centric cross-sectional study in children. Pediatr Allergy Immunol 2007;18(7):566-74.

[8] Penard-Morand C, Charpin D, Raherison C, Kopferschmitt C, Caillaud D, Lavaud F, et al. Long-term exposure to background air pollution related to respiratory and allergic health in schoolchildren. Clin Exp Allergy 2005;35(10):1279-87.

[9] Lee YL, Shaw CK, Su HJ, Lai JS, Ko YC, Huang SL, et al. Climate, traffic-related air pollutants and allergic rhinitis prevalence in middle-school children in Taiwan. Eur Respirat J 2003;21(6):964-70.

[10] Ghunaim N, Wickman M, Almqvist C, Soderstrom L, Ahlstedt S, van Hage M. Sensitization to different pollens and allergic disease in 4-year-old Swedish children. Clin Exp Allergy 2006;36(6):722-7.

[11] Bartkova-Scevkova J. The influence of temperature, relative humidity and rainfall on the occurrence of pollen allergens (Betula, Poaceae, Ambrosia artemisiifolia) in the atmosphere of Bratislava (Slovakia). Int J Biometeorol 2003;48:1-5.

[12] D'Amato G, Liccardi G, Frenguelli G. Thunderstorm-asthma and pollen allergy. Allergy 2007;62(1):11-6.

[13] Unisys Weather Information Systems. Upper air data. URL: http://weather.unisys.com/upper_air/ details.php.

[14] Knorr RS, Condon SK, Dwyer FM, Hoffman DF. Tracking Pediatric Asthma: The Massachusetts Experience Using School Health Records. Environ Health Perspect 2004;112(14):1424-7.

[15] Mandate HOPHSCwS. Early Intervent 2008;36.

[16] Schoenbach V, Rosamond W, editors. Understanding the Fundamentals of Epidemiology: an evolving text. Fall 2000 ed. Chapel Hill, NC: University North Carolina, 2000.

[17] House Bill 1113, The General Assembly of of the Commonwealth of Pennsylvania, 2003 Sess, 2003.

[18] United States Department of Education. Family Educational Rights and Privacy Act (FERPA). Family Policy Compliance Office (FPCO).URL: http://www2.ed.gov/policy/gen/guid/fpco/ferpa/index.html.

[19] Boos D. On generalized score tests. Am Statistician 1992;46:327-33.

[20] Rotnizky A, Jewell N. Hypothesis testing of regression parameters in semiparametric generalized linear models for cluster correlated data. Biometrika 1990;77:485-97.

[21] Mayo Clinic. Humidifiers and Dehumidifiers. Rotnizky A, Jewell N. Hypothesis testing of regression parameters in semiparametric generalized. URL: http://www.mayoclinic.com/health/humidifiers /HQ00076.

[22] American College of Allergy, Asthma, and Immunology (ACAAI). Make Your Child's Room an Allergy-Free Zone. Rotnizky A, Jewell N. Hypothesis testing of regression parameters in semiparametric generalized. URL: http://www.acaai.org/allergist/news/New/Pages/childs-room-allergy-free-zone.aspx.

[23] Logue JN, White MV, Marchetto DJ. Pennsylvania's asthma school project and descriptive pilot investigation: A focus on environmental health tracking. J Environ Health 2007;70(3):21-7.

[24] Vassallo MF, Banerji A, Rudders SA, Clark S, Mullins RJ, Camargo CA. Season of birth and food allergy in children. Ann Allergy Asthma Immunol 2010;104(4):307-13.

In: School, Adolescence and Health Issues
Editors: J. Merrick, A. Tenenbaum and H. A. Omar
ISBN: 978-1-62948-702-1

Chapter 3

SCHOOL-AGE CHILDREN WITH SEVERE HEALTH PROBLEMS

*Cecilia Obeng, PhD**
Department of Applied Health Science, Indiana University,
Bloomington, Indiana, US

ABSTRACT

People living in rural areas in Ghana face impediments to accessing hospitals and clinics. This study examines how culture influences health care–seeking behavior, including the healing processes that participants experience in times of illness, in a Ghana community. The study uses narratives provided by twenty parents about their school-aged children with severe health problems. Results from an analysis of the participants' narratives indicate that participants prefer traditional herbal and/or spiritual 'clinics' to modern clinics/hospitals because of the pleasant relationship established with those healers. Participants also attributed their preference for traditional herbal or spiritual clinics to the low fees charged by the clinics. They noted further that questions about their health problems were always promptly answered at the herbal/spiritual clinics, unlike in modern clinics/hospitals, where they had to wait for hours or days due to delays in releasing laboratory results. However, participants complained about the crowded environment of some of the traditional herbal/spiritual clinics. This study recommends making all traditional clinics patient-friendly in order to expedite healthcare delivery in rural Ghana.

INTRODUCTION

Research on healthcare in Africa indicates that access to healthcare and diagnoses of diseases is difficult on the continent and that many diseases are either misdiagnosed or go untreated (1, 2). In spite of the fact that there has been an improvement in healthcare delivery, especially

* Correspondence: Associate professor Cecilia Obeng, PhD, Department of Applied Health Science, Indiana University, 1025 E 7th Street, HPER 116, Room 296-I, Bloomington, IN 47405 United States. E-mail: cobeng@indiana.edu.

with regard to communicable diseases in the world, communicable diseases are prevalent in Africa (2-4). HIV/AIDS and malaria infection are among the contributing factors associated with a high number of deaths in the region (3, 4). It is also true that a number of sub-Saharan African countries still suffer from some of the worst health problems seen in the world.

The healthcare system in some sub-Saharan African countries is in crisis; maternal and prenatal health problems continue to plague the sub-region. Of all the diseases in the world, 24% are in Africa, with only a few healthcare workers caring for individuals who have health problems (5-7). The shortage of health care workers has had a tremendous impact on the continent. Africa has one of the lowest levels of human resources in the world, and out of the 57countries in which there is a shortage of healthcare workers, 36 of them were in Africa (5-7). Mullan et al. (8) and Callaghan et al. (9) attest to these problems and attribute them to a lack of postgraduate education, retention of graduates after their medical education, coordination between the ministries (education and health), and lack of accreditation of the medical schools in sub-Saharan Africa. The above-mentioned problems, the authors state, have led to a shortage of professionals like doctors, especially, in rural Africa (8, 9).

Scholarship on the shortage of African healthcare workers indicates further that the problem has led to task-shifting in which jobs that should be done by specific professionals in the appropriate health field are assigned to persons with lower qualifications in the field (6). Furthermore, task-shifting is done in Africa to address the healthcare needs (especially with respect to the HIV pandemic that has affected so many lives) on the continent. Job shifting, scholars indicated, will enable well-trained nurses to be involved in prescribing drugs, counselors to help with testing, and some patients to perform certain tasks in their recovering process (9). The main aim of the above-mentioned care system (task-shifting) has been to provide quality care and relieve some of the pressure on healthcare workers (9). The task-shifting idea was explained by the World Health Organization (WHO) in the guidelines in their 2004 publication Integrated Management of Adult and Adolescent Illness and was extended and formalized by WHO/UNAIDS/PEPFAR in 2008 (9). A report by WHO indicates further that only 1% of the world's funding allocated for health care goes to Africa. It is well known that Africans suffer from high levels of malnutrition (10), the problems of which are attributed to protein energy deficiency (10). Infertility and premature death are also unnecessarily high in some of these regions (11).

Given the unfortunate state of the healthcare situation described above, this study examined 20 narratives of parents in rural Africa (Ghana) in order to understand the healthcare–seeking behavior of the participants. Also examined were the various stages that parents have undergone to find care for their children's health issues.

Our study

This study was approved by the Institutional Review Board of Indiana University's Human Subjects Committee. The population for this study was comprised of 20 participants who visited five traditional clinics in a rural area in Ghana. Participants were interviewed by the principal investigator and two paid research assistants. The research assistants had lived in the school district for over twenty years. The research assistants contacted approximately 30 potential parents for interviews for this study. Four people were not able to participate because of conflicts with their schedules. Twenty out of the 26 qualified for this study because they had children with severe health problems and chronic health diseases, and the parents were also happy to be part of the study. The instrument used in the study consisted of both closed-ended and open-ended questions. The closed-ended questions concerned the demographic information of participants. The open-ended questions were used as the main questions for this qualitative study. The open-ended questions asked participants to narrate their reason(s) for attending herbal/spiritual clinics. Participation was voluntary, and consent was given before parents participated in interviews. In order to verify whether what participants reported was an accurate representation of their views, the researchers returned after 10 days and reviewed with participants what they had reported during the first visit.

Coding and data analysis

Two people (the principal investigator and a volunteer colleague) were involved in the coding of the completed questionnaires for this study, Health Care Seeking Avenues of Parents of School-Aged Children with Severe Health Problems in a Community in Ghana. The coding involved an assessment of the narratives and the content of the data (by the coders) with the intent of identifying common themes.

A qualitative analysis was conducted on the responses to the open-ended questions collected during the interviews. Responses were grouped into themes for the purpose of analysis.

FINDINGS

The results are organized into and discussed under the following themes: 1) demographic information of participants and 2) participants' narratives about their visits to traditional clinics.

Demographic information

As drawn from the parents' narratives, their children were aged between seven and seventeen years. Participants' children lived in four different villages approximately eighty-five miles from the capital, Accra, in Ghana. Sixteen of the children whose parents were interviewed lived with both of their biological parents. Four girls lived with their grandparents (mothers' parents). Eight of the children attended school, which was almost two miles away from their homes. The other 12 children were in schools close to their homes at the time of this study. Parents reported their children had asthma, kwashiorkor, epilepsy, and diabetes. The table 1 below details information about the participants.

Table 1. Information about the participants

Participants	Age of Parents	Sex of Parents	No. of Children	School Attended	No. of Visits to a Government Hospital or Clinic	No. of Visits to a Traditional Clinic	Kind of Diseases Reported
Parent 1	50	M	9	Public	2	20 or more	Epilepsy
Parent2	45	F	8	Public	1	Many times	Asthma
Parent 3	43	F	6	Public	2	Over 15 times	Asthma
Parent 4	43	M	7	Pubic	2	Over 15times	Asthma
Parent 5	42	F	7	public	2	Over 10 times	Asthma
Parent 6	41	F	6	Public	0	Over 15 times	Kwashiorkor
Parent 7	41	F	6	Public	0	Over 15 times	Kwashiorkor
Parent 8	40	F	6	Public	1	10	Kwashiorkor
Parent 9	40	F	7	Public	1	Over 15 times	Kwashiorkor
Parent 10	39	F	6	Public	0	Over 15 times	Kwashiorkor
Parent 11	38	F	8	Public	3	Over 20 times	Diabetes
Parent 12	38	M	9	Public	5	Over 15 times	Epilepsy,
Parent 13	35	F	4	Public	3	10	Asthma
Parent 14	25	F	2	Private	4	Over 15 times	Diabetes
Parent 15	23	F	1	Private	2	Over 15 times	Asthma
Parent 16	22	F	1	Public	6	Over 20 times	Asthma
Parent 17	22	F	1	Public	2	Over 15 times	Asthma
Parent 18	21	F	1	Public	1	10	Kwashiorkor
Parent 19	21	F	1	Public	2	Over 15 times	Asthma
Parent 20	20	F	1	Public	1	10	Kwashiorkor

Participants and their narratives

Thematic summaries of participants' narratives are given below. Six participants, one male and five females, reported that a lack of money to send their children to government hospitals/clinics contributed to their decision to send their children to traditional clinics. One participant wrote:

> "We decided to take him to an herbal/spiritual clinic because we had tried several times to save money towards sending him to the hospital but we had not been able to save enough money to afford transportation cost to go to the nearest clinic which is twenty miles away. I think to send him to the hospital, which is about eight-five miles, would have been a lifetime's saving and we couldn't have waited that long given the severity of the illness."

Five of the participants, aged between 21 and 43 years, said that the money that the traditional clinics charge patients motivated them to send their children to traditional clinics. One of the participants who sent his child to a traditional clinic wrote:

> "The day that our family was informed about the herbal clinic was the best day for our family. The money that the healer's clinic charged was just about one-hundredth of what our friends told us it would have cost at the government hospital."

Five participants, all female, said the friendly environment of the traditional clinics motivated them to send their children to the traditional clinic. A participant wrote:

> "Our herbalist/spiritualist doctor was friendly and spent many hours with us. He and his assistant answered all our questions. We understand that in the Western-based clinics the maximum amount of time that the physician can have for you was twenty minutes. The many questions our family had could not have been answered within the twenty-minutes time period let alone the doctors' twenty minutes maximum time frame."

A mother said:

> "The Herbal/ spiritual clinics is the best place for those of us who do not have time to wait for a whole day. I understand some of the tests could take a week or even a whole year for the doctor to tell you the cause of your illness. Also, I understand if you are not lucky they will just say they do not know the cause of your illness. I like the herbal clinic because of their efficient work ethic but the many materials in the herbal clinic made me uncomfortable and added to my stress level."

Four mothers reported that they went to an herbalist clinic because the herbalists were able to answer their questions concerning their children's illnesses. One mother reported:

> "We got all the answers that we suspected were causing the illness from the herbalist and we now know the best place to go when anybody in our family is sick. Our only problem was the many 'materials' that were in the clinic also the place was filthy."

Another mother said:

> "The herbalist and his assistant were patient and answered all our many question but my biggest problem was that there was no space for us to sit in the clinic, the clinic was cluttered with materials and the place was also dirty."

DISCUSSION

Most of the participants' narratives suggested that the first-rate performance of the work done by traditional healers encouraged them to choose those healers over Western-trained physicians. Specifically, we learned of a better work ethic and a more intimate working relationship between the traditional care-givers and their clients. The low charges prompt answers given to patients' families about the causative agents of their diseases, excellent working relationships between the caregivers and their clients, and effective care at the traditional clinics was convincing of better treatment for the participants.

From their narratives, it was obvious that the traditional clinics were cluttered with the materials they used in their profession, thereby posing a hindrance or potential danger to easy patient movement and, consequently, making it difficult for patients and the healers to find much needed space. This also created unsanitary conditions in the clinics, according to participants narratives.

This study recommends improvements to achieve patient-friendly and hygienic environments in the form of better sanitation and de-cluttering of unwanted materials from the healing sites/clinics of the traditional healers in order to ensure optimal efficiency. This recommendation is motivated by the fact that participants believed that improvements in the environments of some of the traditional healers would ease their stress and improve their health when they are at these sites.

Limitations and future research

Although using twenty participants' experiences from five clinics for this study may appear limiting, it represents more than two-thirds of the traditional clinics in the research site. Also, we were aware of the dangerous possibility of our personal judgments intervening in their narratives. Being aware of these potential pitfalls helped, however, to mitigate them. Specifically, our awareness of this unique situation kept us on guard against intervening in the telling of participants' narratives. In the future, and based upon the fact that participants wanted improvement in the traditional clinic setting, a survey will be done to determine whether there have been improvements (structural and interactional) enacted by healers in order to enhance their profession.

REFERENCES

[1] Petti CA, Polage CR, Quinn TC, et al. Laboratory medicine in Africa: A barrier to effective health care. Clinical Infectious Diseases. 2006;42:377-82.

[2] Dacombe RJ, Squire SB, Ramsav ARC, Banda HT, Bates I. Essential medical Laboratory Services: their role in delivering equitable health care in Malawi. Malawi Med J 2006:18(2):77-9.

[3] Joint United Nations Programme on HIV/AIDS. 2011. URL: http://www.unaids.org/en/media/unaids/contentassets/documents/unaidspublication/2011/JC2216_WorldAIDSday_report_2011_en.pdf.

[4] World Malaria Report. 2011. URL: http://www.who.int/malaria/world_malaria_ report_2011/WHOGMP_burden_estimates_qa.pdf.

[5] The World Health Organization. 2006. URL:who.int/gho/publications/ world_health_statistics/whostat2006_10highlights.pdf.

[6] WHO/UNAIDS/PEPFAR. Task Shifting: Global Recommendations and Guidelines. Geneva. 2008. URL: http://www.who.int/healthsystems/task_ shifting/en/index.html.

[7] Health Poverty Action. URL: http://healthpovertyaction.org/policy-and-resources/health-systems/the-global-shortage-of-health-workers/.

[8] Mullan F, Freyhwot S, Omaswa F, Wassermann T. Medical schools in sub-Saharan Africa. Lancet 2011;377:1113-21.

[9] Callaghan M, Ford N, Schneider H. A systematic review of task-shifting for HIV treatment and care in Africa. Hum Resources Health 2010;8:8.

[10] Maletnlema TN. Hunger and malnutrition: The determinant of development: the case for Africa and its food and nutrition workers. East Afr Med J 1992;69(8):424-7.

[11] Amico P, Aran C, Avila C. HIV Spending as a Share of Total Health Expenditure: An Analysis of Regional Variation in a Multi-Country Study. 2010 PLoS ONE 5(9): e12997. doi:10.1371/journal.pone.0012997

In: School, Adolescence and Health Issues
Editors: J. Merrick, A. Tenenbaum and H. A. Omar
ISBN: 978-1-62948-702-1

Chapter 4

PREDICTING PEDIATRICIAN SICK VISITS FOR ADOLESCENTS

Laura Nabors, PhD, ABPP* and Brian T Olsen, MA
Counseling Program, Department of Health and Human Services, College of Education, Criminal Justice, Health and Human Services and Department of Psychology, University of Cincinnati, Cincinnati, Ohio, US

ABSTRACT

The purpose of the current study was to examine factors related to adolescents seeking medical care when feeling ill. Over 400 high school-age students participated. Adolescents provided self-report data. A regression model was used to examine predictors related to adolescent reports of visiting their doctor when ill. Adolescents were more likely to seek care if they believed their provider had a caring attitude. Adolescents who tended to treat their symptoms with over-the-counter remedies were less likely to seek care when they were ill. Future studies should consider family, contextual, and individual level barriers that prevent adolescents from seeking care when they are ill.

INTRODUCTION

Adolescents often forego health care or lack access to needed health care (1-3). More information is needed about factors related to foregoing care. Foregoing health care may be especially important for adolescents, who are apt to engage in risky behaviors (e.g., alcohol use) that are important to discuss with their pediatricians (4). The current study contributes to the literature by providing information on factors related to ignoring symptoms and seeking health care from their doctor when they are ill. Klein et al. (5) reported that about one-third of the adolescents in their study had missed needed healthcare. This study examined factors

* Correspondence: Laura Nabors, Counseling Program, Department of Health and Human Services, College of Education, Criminal Justice, Health and Human Services, Box 0068, Cincinnati, OH 45221-0376, United States. E-mail: naborsla@ucmail.uc.edu.

related to adolescents' tendency to ignore their symptoms, which can be a risk factor for receiving healthcare when they are ill. Besides ignoring, taking over-the-counter (OTC) medications to relieve symptoms or cure them may be a way for adolescents to avoid going to see their doctor when they are ill (6, 7). Adolescents also may be more likely to see their pediatrician if they feel that he or she has "caring" attitude, which reflects on their having a positive relationship with their pediatrician (8). For the current study, a logistic regression analysis was used to examine the relations among self-medicating by going to the drugstore to get medicine, ignoring symptoms, opinions about the doctor's attitude, and going to see a primary care doctor when ill.

OUR STUDY

Four hundred and thirty-five adolescents (271 females and 164 males) completed surveys. The adolescents were in high school and ranged between 14 and 18 years of age (M = 15 years, SD = 1 year, 3 months). A university-based institutional review board approved this study. Parent consent and child assent were used for youth between the ages of 14 and 17 years. Adolescents who were 18 years old provided consent for study participation.

Students provided data during health classes, completing a survey developed by Nabors et al. (9). This study was approved by our institution's university-based institutional review board.

FINDINGS

Fifty-eight percent (n = 251) of these adolescents indicated that they typically go to a primary care doctor when they are ill. Forty-one percent (n = 179) reported going to a drugstore when ill and 34% (n = 147) reported that they ignored their symptoms when feeling ill. Ninety-four percent (n = 406) reported that they valued the characteristic of caring as a valuable trait for a doctor.

Variables in our logistic regression model were centered prior to conducting our analyses. The best fit model included the three aforementioned variables (going to the drugstore to get medicine, ignoring symptoms, opinions about the doctor having a caring attitude) and their two 2-way interaction terms. The chi-square for our final model was significant ($X2 = 87.99$, $df = 5$, $p < .001$) indicating that the set of variables improved the prediction of the log odds. Our model predicted 25% of the variance in the dependent variable (Nagelkerke $R2 = .25$; see Table 1).

Follow-up regression models were used to examine the significant interaction of ignoring symptoms and caring attitude of the pediatrician. Results indicated that participants reporting they did not ignore their symptoms were almost 5 times more likely to go to see a private doctor if they valued a caring attitude, $X2\ (1) = 6.92$, $p =.009$ ($B = 1.589$, $SE = .627$, Wald Statistic = 6.421). This variable predicted 3% of the variance in going to the doctor when ill. The second regression model did not yield significant results, indicating that caring attitude was not related to ignoring symptoms.

Table 1. Variables predicting going to a private physician when feeling ill

Variables	*B*	*SE*	*Wald Statistic*	*df*	*p*	*Exp(B)*
Caring Attitude	1.129	.478	5.571	1	.018	3.092
OTC Meds	-.466	.227	4.191	1	.041	.628
Ignore	-1.539	.235	43.032	1	.001	.215
Caring x Ignore	1.895	.931	4.143	1	.042	6.655
Caring x OTC Meds	.625	.984	.403	1	.526	1.868

Next, we examined the interaction of ignoring symptoms and purchasing OTC medications to treat symptoms. The regression model for adolescents who did ignore symptoms and went to the drugstore for medicine was significant, X2 (1) = 5.922, p = .015 (B = .928, SE = .381, Wald Statistic = 5.392). Adolescents who ignored their symptoms were 2.5 times more likely to purchase OTC medicines; ignoring predicted 5.5% of the variance in purchase of OTC medicines. Participants who reported they did not ignore their symptoms were less likely to go get OTC medicines when they were not feeling well, X2 (1) = 21.45, p < .001 (B = - 1.229, SE = .274, Wald Statistic = 20.137); and being less likely to go to the drugstore predicted 10% of the variance in not ignoring symptoms.

DISCUSSION

Study findings provided information for pediatricians and other health professionals who provide medical care for adolescents, who represent a group that often has limited access to health services (1, 2, 5). Similar to other research (7), our results revealed that participants who purchased over-the-counter medications were likely to ignore their symptoms and not seek care. Pediatricians could ask adolescents about use of OTC medicines to self-treat, so that they do not need to visit a doctor. This screening question could identify adolescents who would benefit from discussing reasons to schedule a visit with their doctors and education about problems related to ignoring medical symptoms. Consistent with the literature [8] findings of this study also showed that for adolescents, who tended not to ignore their symptoms, perceiving their doctors to be caring was related to seeing their pediatrician when ill. Thus, showing caring reaches those likely to come for appointments.

More information is needed about why some adolescents do not visit their pediatrician, given that we predicted 25% of the variance in our dependent variable. Exploration of other variables, such as perceptions of pediatricians' competence, might better explain why adolescents do not access care. Data for this research reflected adolescents' self-report and reports may not reflect adolescents' behaviors. Analyzing show rates for appointments would provide objective data to check actual attendance at the doctors' offices. Future research should focus on addressing barriers to receiving care based on a lack of insurance and transportation issues, which are other factors that may prohibit adolescents from seeking care when they are ill.

ACKNOWLEDGEMENTS

We would like to thank the University of Cincinnati for supporting our research efforts.

REFERENCES

[1] Committee on Adolescence. Achieving quality health services for adolescents. Pediatrics 2008;121:1263-70.
[2] Society for Adolescent Medicine. Access to health care for adolescents and young adults. J Adolesc Health 2004;35:342-4.
[3] Vinner R, McFarlane A. Provision of age appropriate health services for young people has been ignored. BMJ 2000;321:1022.
[4] Klein JD, Wilson KM. Delivering quality care: Adolescents' discussion of health risks with their providers. J Adolesc Health 2002;30:190-5.
[5] Klein JD, Wilson KM, McNulty M, et al. Access to medical care for adolescents: Results from the 1997 Commonwealth Fund Survey of the health of adolescent girls. J Adolesc Health 1999;25:120-30.
[6] Gray NJ, Cantrill JA, Noyce PR. Health repertories: an understanding of lay management of minor ailments. Patient Educ Couns 2002;47: 237-44.
[7] Thompson WM, Poulton R. Medications taken by 26-year-olds. Intern Med J 2002;32:305-10.
[8] Pommier J, Mouchtouris A, Billot L, et al. Self-reported determinants of health service use by French adolescents. Int J Adolesc Med Health 2001;13:115-29.
[9] Nabors LA, Lehmkuhl HD, Parkins IS, & Drury AM. Reading about over-the-counter medications. Issues Compr Pediatr Nurs 2004;27:297-305.

In: School, Adolescence and Health Issues
Editors: J. Merrick, A. Tenenbaum and H. A. Omar
ISBN: 978-1-62948-702-1

Chapter 5

SCHOOL CLIMATE AND PSYCHOLOGICAL HARDINESS AMONG ADOLESCENTS

Jagpreet Kaur, PhD, MSc, MEd, PGDCA** *and Kulwinder Singh, PhD, MPhil, MA, BSc

Department of Education, Punjabi University, Patiala, India

ABSTRACT

In this chapter we examine the impact of school climate on psychological hardiness of creative adolescents. A descriptive method of research was used for the conduct of the present study with a random sample of 1,011 Indian adolescents. Several standardized tools were employed: Psychological Hardiness Scale, Test of Creative Thinking and School Organizational Climate Description Questionnaire (SOCDQ). Creative adolescents were found to possess significantly higher level of psychological hardiness and its dimensions than their non-creative counterparts. Also, significant differences were found in commitment, challenge and psychological hardiness among adolescents related to different types of school climate. Further, creative adolescents within an autonomous type of school climate were found to possess significantly higher control upon them and those with controlled climate were hardier as compared to their non-creative counterparts belonging to other types of school climate. However, school climate does not seem to affect the commitment and challenge dimensions of psychological hardiness among creative adolescents. The paper calls for intervention efforts to be made not only to nurture children's creativity and enhancing their psychological hardiness, but also for promoting conducive school climate.

* Correspondence: Jagpreet Kaur, Lecturer, PhD, MSc, MEd, PGDCA, Department of Education, Arts Block 5, Punjabi University, Patiala (PB)-147002, India. E-mail: jagpreetmahal@yahoo.com.

INTRODUCTION

Education in a free, dynamic society aims at helping each and every member of that society to develop fully their capacity, talents and to learn to utilize them creatively and continuously to improve themselves and society. The major goal of education is to ensure excellence in every aspect of life by continuously improving the quality and relevance of every aspect of education. Thus, the school as a formal agency of education has certain goals that include intellectual (usually referred as academic goals) and practical goals concerned with meaningful living in a complex society. Children grow up in several environments. Home, school, and community are the setting for social and intellectual experiences from which they acquire and develop the skills, attitudes and attachments which characterize them as individuals and shape their choice and performance of adult roles (1).

Psychological hardiness – as a combination of adaptive personality traits that allows one to overcome stressful life-events – has emerged as an important variable in psychological researches in the previous two decades. Hardiness personality style has been proposed as a source of positive resistance to the debilitating effects of stressful life events on health (2). The hardy personality is a constellation of three important personality traits: commitment, control, and challenge. Hardy persons tend to have dedication to a purpose, a sense of control over events, and tend to perceive events as opportunities and challenges rather than stressors. Hardy persons were presented as having considerable curiosity and tending to find their experiences interesting and meaningful (3). They believe they can be influential through what they imagine, say and do. They accept change to be the norm, and regard it as the key to development.

Specifically, hardy individuals were found to be high in commitment. That is, they showed a tendency to involve them in, rather than experience alienation from, whatever they were doing or encountering. They showed a positive response to challenge. They believed that change rather than stability was normal in life. They appraised change as an interesting incentive to personal growth, not as a threat to security. Also, hardy individuals perceived to have a high level of control over their lives. They felt and behaved as though they were influential rather than helpless in facing the various rewards and punishments of life. Psychologically hardy people tend to have an internal locus of control (3).

Review of related literature provides a picture depicting psychological hardiness - an emerging area of research in personality - to be affecting not only ill or stress prone individuals, but also to contribute to mental health and well-being in various population groups, namely, adolescents/youth, professionals, patients suffering from chronic diseases as well as elderly persons. Psychological hardiness was found to be facilitative of enhanced performance among students, both in academic and non-academic aspects of achievement (4-8). Also, psychological hardiness was found to contribute to better quality of life among old age people (9-14). Psychological hardiness has been reported to act as a buffer in reducing stress among different professional groups and is a catalyst to better mental health (15-19). Another group of researchers found psychological hardiness to be facilitative in restoring mental and physical health among chronic patients suffering from different kinds of physical ailments (20-23). Another important fact found was that successful people in different careers exhibit higher levels of psychological hardiness as compared to non-successful people, thereby indicating a positive relationship between psychological hardiness and success in different life situations (19, 24-27).

During childhood and adolescence most of the social influences upon individual can be categorized as being associated either with home or with school climate. In the early years the family is the most potent source of influence, but once children have entered school, new opportunities are created for adults, and for peers and older pupils to influence individual development. The function of the school is to socialize, and education is a process of growth. In fact, the school may be defined as an agency designed to provide the resources, activities and guidance necessary to help each child discover and actualize his potential. It presents the child with a planned environment with most of the activities controlled, not rigidly, but a sort of regulated permissiveness (28). Thus, the school must be looked upon as a force secondary in importance only to the home in the development of human personality. Nevertheless, the school's role as a shaper of personality is formidable. The school climate has a marked influence on the student's emotional states and, through them, on his personality. The student, as child and adolescent, spends many years in an educational environment. The wholesome school climate is often adequate to counteract any unfavourable emotional patterns of behaviours established in the home.

The wholesome climate of the school has a therapeutic effect on his personality. An adolescent's school experiences exert a potent influence on his developing personality pattern. The school shares with the home the responsibility of helping a young person achieve those behaviour characteristics that can ensure for him the making of satisfactory adjustments to the demands on him of the various areas of his present and future life activities. All the characteristics, which constitute the personality of the adolescent, offer it in unique combinations to be explained in terms of individual differences as measured by certain constellations in the personality pattern – both cognitive and affective. The intellectual development has a specific role in shaping of a personality and creativity is the key element in this area.

Creativity has been considered in terms of process, product or person (29) and has been defined as the interpersonal and intrapersonal process by means of which original, high quality, and genuinely significant products are developed. In dealing with young children, the focus should be on the process, i.e., developing and generating original ideas, which is seen as the basis of creative potential. When trying to understand this process, it is helpful to consider it as a differentiation between convergent and divergent thought (30). Problems associated with convergent thought often have one correct solution. But problems associated with divergent thought require the problem-solver to generate many solutions, a few of which will be novel, of high quality, and workable--hence creative. Creativity is the ability to see things in a new way, to see problems that no one else may even realize exist, and then come up with new, unique, and effective solutions to these problems. Creativity has been theorized as one of the dimensions of cluster three traits of giftedness, the other two being : average, general or specific abilities and task commitment (31).

Creativity of a person depends on his environment. The more congenial the environment for creativity, the more a person is likely to exhibit his creativity (32-39). While the creative may have been more talented to begin with, it also looks as if their home environment assisted in the flowering of their creativity. Our environment shapes, though it does not determine, our creativity in various ways. A punitive environment can instill in us much fearfulness and blockage. On the other hand a cultural or family environment that encourages risk taking or experimentation may stimulate a strong pioneering or innovative effort. Environment not only shapes personality, it may also influence the person having or not having various creativity-related abilities. Besides shaping one's personality and ability, the environment may block or facilitate creative activities.

It has been revealed that students of central schools are more creative than those of private schools (34). In another study, it was found that convent school children to be more creative than the traditional school children (40). It was also concluded that creativity have modest associations with perceptions of family and school climates (37). School climate has been found to have a positive effect on student creativity and achievement (32-33, 41-48). Also, it has been found to have a positive bearing on personality development among adolescent students (49-55, 48). Creativeness has been found to have a relationship with school type (34, 40 56- 57)

In adolescence, the thrust towards development of identity, social and individual needs for independence and individuation and adaptation to the increased richness of experiences are all factors in the development of creativity. One can be creative if the awareness and expression of inner life are encouraged or favored by parents and the interests are permitted to develop at its own pace. In some families children are given considerable freedom even at an early age, to explore the world around them and make decisions. Such type of socio-psychological environment helps children grow creatively. The development of creativity appears to be enhanced by certain dimensions in the life of the child. These dimensions are: (a) An open environment, (b) the active use of creative skills, (c) a result of previous knowledge, and (d) a disciplined use of technique. In fact child's creativity can take place only in free environment where his imagination is given a chance of free play (32-36).

However, psychological hardiness among gifted adolescents, especially the creatives has been less explored, though it has been studied in relation to a number of cognitive and non-cognitive variables. School climate is a major area affecting the adolescent's personality development in a unique way. Moreover, the focus on gifted adolescents and their personality development in the present highly industrialized, competitive, and challenging era, where school conditions and family life, too are undergoing a sea change calls for the attention of researchers. There is paucity of research on effects of school climate on creative development as well as personality formation among adolescents. Hence, it was thought worthwhile to explore the impact of school climate on psychological hardiness among creatively gifted adolescents.

OUR STUDY

The population of the study was the secondary school students studying in 1,151 government secondary schools situated in 17 districts (now 20) in Punjab state of India. The number of schools in each district in Punjab varies from 23 in Mansa to 145 in Ludhiana. Keeping in view, the uneven location of schools in the districts, two districts each were selected randomly from three clusters of districts having highest, average and lowest number of schools. Further, selection of schools from each of these six randomly selected districts was made on random basis giving due weightage to boys and girls schools situated in urban and rural areas. A total of 44 government schools were randomly selected for the conduct of the present study. A total number of 350 teachers teaching secondary classes in these government secondary schools were included in the sample to seek their perceptions on school climate. A sample of 30-45 adolescents from each of the selected school, totaling 1011 adolescents (male = 448 and female = 563; mean age = 17 years) was taken for assessment of creative talent and psychological hardiness. We used the following research tools:

- The Psychological Hardiness Scale (59) was used for measuring psychological hardiness among adolescents. This is a 30-item scale having 17 positively worded and 13 negatively worded statements, to be responded on 5-point rating i.e., strongly agree [1], agree [2], neither agree nor disagree [3], disagree [4] and strongly disagree [5]. The scale has 10 items each pertaining to challenge, control, and commitment dimensions. The scoring in case of positively worded statements is from "5 to 1" from 'strongly agree' to 'strongly disagree' and vice versa in case of negatively worded statements. The scale provides three dimensional scores and a composite score as psychological hardiness score. The range of score in the dimensions is 10-50 and 30-150 for total hardiness score; and high score is indicative of strong presence of challenge, control, and commitment and being a hardy individual.
- A verbal test of creative thinking was used to classify adolescents in terms of being creative and non-creative (58). The test contains certain primary traits as has been described by Guilford related to divergent thinking which seem to go with creative output. The verbal test of creative thinking consists of four activities, namely, consequences test, unusual uses test, similarity test, and product improvement test. The dimensional scores obtained from each of the test activities are fluency, flexibility and originality. The summated scores on these abilities have been taken as composite verbal creativity scores.
- The School Organizational Climate Description Questionnaire (60) was used to classify selected senior secondary schools in terms of being: (i) open, (ii) autonomous, (iii) familiar, (iv) controlled, (v) paternal, and (vi) closed climate.

All the teachers teaching secondary classes in the school concerned were administered the School Organizational Climate Description Questionnaire (SOCDQ) for the classification of schools in terms of six types of school climate, namely open, autonomous, familiar, controlled, paternal to closed. This classification of schools was made on the basis of scores of teachers on eight sub-tests in the School Organizational Climate Description Questionnaire (SOCDQ) by a double standardization procedure (ipsative and normative) with a mean of 50 and standard deviation of 10. The assessment of creative talent was carried out by the verbal tests of creative thinking. After identification of creative and non-creative students (based on third and first quartile respectively), the psychological hardiness scale was administered.

For studying the effect of school climate in terms of being open, autonomous, familiar, controlled, paternal and closed on psychological hardiness and its dimensions among creative adolescents, 2 x 6 factorial design was thought worth while. The distribution of high and low creative adolescents in terms of six types of school climate obtained on the basis of 1011 Indian adolescents is provided in the table 1. It is evident from the table I that number of students was fixed in terms of six types of school climate.

Table 1. Distribution of adolescents in six types of school climate

S. No.	Type of School Climate	Creativity (A)		
		High Creative (A_1)	Low Creative (A_2)	Total
1.	Open (B_1)	52	52	104
2.	Autonomous (B_2)	27	43	70
3.	Familiar (B_3)	51	43	94
4.	Controlled (B_4)	58	49	107
5.	Paternal (B_5)	26	29	55
6.	Closed (B_6)	65	51	116

Table 2. Summary of ANOVA (creativity x school climate): Psychological hardiness and its dimensions

S. No.	Dimension of Psychological Hardiness	Source of Variation	SS	df	MS	F
1.	Commitment	Creativity (A)	161.94	1	161.4	141.90**
		School climate(B)	131.3	5	26.3	2.30*
		A x B	54.1	5	10.8	0.98
		Within	3286.6	288	11.4	
		Total	5091.4	299		
2.	Control	Creativity (A)	3346.7	1	3346.7	229.03**
		School climate (B)	96.8	5	19.4	1.32
		A X B	158.3	5	31.7	2.17*
		Within	4208.4	288	14.6	
		Total	7810.2	299		
3.	Challenge	Creativity (A)	5410.3	1	5410.3	245.69**
		School climate (B)	376.2	5	75.2	3.42*
		A X B	210.1	5	42.0	1.91
		Within	6342.0	288	22.0	
		Total	12338.5	299		
4.	Psychological Hardiness	Creativity (A)	29462	1	29462	657.70**
		School climate(B)	1172	5	234	5.23**
		A X B	593	5	119	2.65*
		Within	12901	288	45	
		Total	44128	299		

** $p < .01$, * $p < .05$.

FINDINGS

The significance of mean differences across high and low levels of creativity and six types of school climate and their interaction effect on psychological hardiness and its dimensions was tested by applying two-way analysis of variance. The results are given in table 2.

The perusal of table 2 reveals that the main effect of creativity was shown be significant for commitment, control, challenge dimensions of hardiness as well as global hardiness (F = 141.90, 229.03, 245.69, 657.70; p<.01), indicating that the creative adolescents are significantly more committed, possess greater control upon themselves and have more challenge-accepting tendency and are more hardy than their non-creative counterparts. Further, the main effect of school climate turned out to be significant for commitment and challenge dimensions of hardiness as well as for global hardiness (F = 2.30, 3.42; p<.05, 5.23; p<.01), thereby meaning that adolescents belonging to different types of school climate differ significantly on commitment and challenge dimensions of psychological hardiness as well as global hardiness.

Further, it can be observed from the table 2 that the interaction effect of creativity and school climate was shown to be non-significant for the commitment and challenge dimensions of hardiness (F = 0.98, 1.91; p<.05), indicating that the significant main effects of creativity and school climate are independent of each other to explain commitment and challenge dimensions of psychological hardiness among adolescents. As may be seen from table 3, creative adolescents have significantly higher commitment and challenge scores than their non-creative counterparts irrespective of the type of school climate.

Table 3. Mean and SD of commitment dimension of psychological hardiness among adolescents in creativity x school climate factorial design

Type of School Climate		**Creativity (A)**		**Total Mean**
		Creative (A_1)	**Non-creative (A_2)**	
Open (B_1)	Mean	31.84	27.80	29.82
	SD	2.17	4.14	
Autonomous (B_2)	Mean	33.80	28.00	30.90
	SD	3.64	3.69	
Familiar (B_3)	Mean	32.92	29.64	31.28
	SD	2.98	3.97	
Controlled (B_4)	Mean	33.40	28.16	30.78
	SD	3.06	4.10	
Paternal (B_5)	Mean	32.36	28.04	30.20
	SD	3.78	2.76	
Closed (B_6)	Mean	31.96	26.76	29.36
	SD	2.89	2.67	
Total Mean		32.71	28.07	

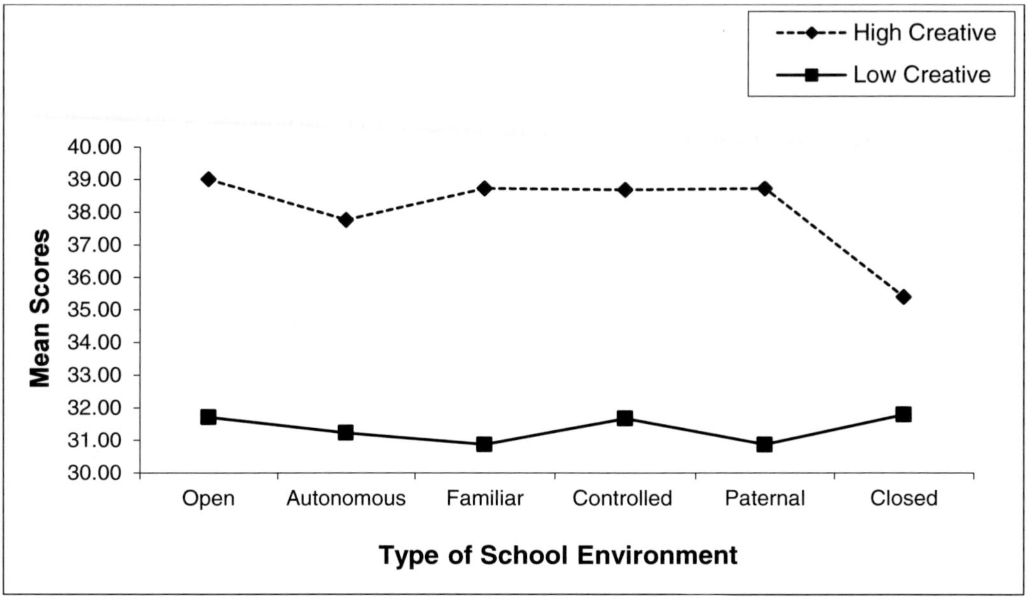

Figure 1. Interactive effect of creativity and school climate on control dimension of psychological hardiness.

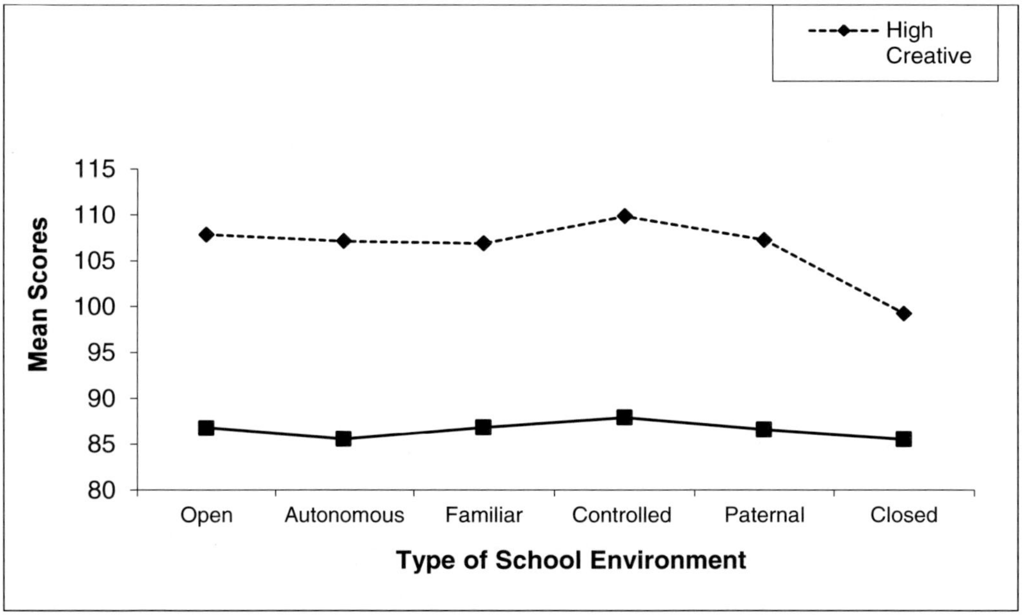

Figure 2. Interactive effect of creativity and school climate on psychological hardiness.

It is evident from the table 3 that creative adolescents within an autonomous type of school climate have highest mean commitment score (33.80) as compared to their counterparts with open (31.84), familiar (32.92) controlled (33.40), paternal (32.36) and closed (31.96) type of school climate. Also, the perusal of table V reveals that creative adolescents with controlled type of school climate have significantly higher mean challenge scores (37.76) as compared to their counterparts with open (37.00), autonomous (35.56), familiar (35.24) paternal (36.16) and closed (31.88) type of school climate. It is worth nothing here that creative adolescents with closed type of school climate scored lowest on the challenge dimension of psychological hardiness. (31.88).

Table 4. Mean and SD of control dimension of psychological hardiness among adolescents in creativity x school climate factorial design

Type of School Climate (B)		Creativity (A) Creative (A_1)	Non-creative (A_2)	Total Mean
Open (B_1)	Mean	39.00	31.72	35.36
	SD	2.83	4.50	
Autonomous (B_2)	Mean	37.76	31.24	34.50
	SD	3.29	4.02	
Familiar (B_3)	Mean	38.72	30.88	34.80
	SD	3.12	4.63	
Controlled (B_4)	Mean	38.68	31.68	35.18
	SD	4.98	3.39	
Paternal (B_5)	Mean	38.72	30.88	34.80
	SD	4.07	3.87	
Closed (B_6)	Mean	35.40	31.80	33.60
	SD	2.33	3.96	
Total Mean		38.05	31.37	

The table 4 shows that creative adolescents within an open type of school climate have significantly higher mean control scores (39.00) as compared to their counterparts with autonomous (37.76), familiar (38.72), controlled (38.68), paternal (38.72) and closed (35.40) type of school climate. It is worth noting here that creative adolescents with a closed type of school climate scored lowest on control dimension of psychological hardiness (35.40).

Table 5. Mean and SD of challenge dimension of psychological hardiness among adolescents in creativity x school climate factorial design

Type of School Climate (B)		Creativity (A) Creative (A_1)	Non-creative (A_2)	Total Mean
Open (B_1)	Mean	37.00	27.24	
	SD	2.08	3.26	32.12
Autonomous (B_2)	Mean	35.56	26.32	
	SD	3.86	4.82	30.94
Familiar (B_3)	Mean	35.24	26.32	
	SD	4.70	3.85	30.78
Controlled (B_4)	Mean	37.76	28.08	
	SD	8.70	4.56	32.92
Paternal (B_5)	Mean	36.16	27.68	
	SD	5.46	4.56	31.92
Closed (B_6)	Mean	31.88	27.00	
	SD	3.80	3.57	29.44
Total Mean		35.60	27.11	

Further, the perusal of the table II reveals that the interaction effect of creativity and school climate is significant for control dimension of psychological hardiness as well as global hardiness ($F = 2.17, 2.65; p<.05$), indicating that the significant main effect of creativity is dependent upon the non-significant main effect of school climate to explain the control dimension of hardiness as well as global hardiness among adolescents (figure 1 and 2).

Table 6. Mean and SD of psychological hardiness among adolescents in creativity x school climate factorial design

Type of School Climate (B)		Creativity (A)		Total Mean
		Creative (A_1)	Non-creative (A_2)	
Open (B_1)	Mean	107.84	86.76	97.30
	SD	4.73	6.53	
Autonomous (B_2)	Mean	107.12	85.56	96.34
	SD	6.06	3.79	
Familiar (B_3)	Mean	106.88	86.84	96.86
	SD	5.85	5.37	
Controlled (B_4)	Mean	109.84	87.92	98.88
	SD	11.63	7.59	
Paternal (B_5)	Mean	107.24	86.60	96.92
	SD	8.68	6.72	
Closed (B_6)	Mean	99.24	85.56	92.40
	SD	5.39	4.01	
Total Mean		106.36	86.54	

It can be observed from table 6 that creative adolescents within a controlled type of school climate have the highest level of psychological hardiness (109.84) as compared to their counterparts with open (107.84), autonomous (107.12), familiar (106.88) paternal (107.24) and closed (9.24) type of school climate. It may also be noted from the table 5 that creative adolescents belonging to a closed type of school climate scored lowest on psychological hardiness (99.24).

DISCUSSION

The results of the study revealed that creative adolescents are more committed, have greater control over themselves, along with more challenge-accepting tendency and are hardier than their non-creative counterparts. So, the creative talent at secondary school stage need to be nurtured as the fuller use of creative and hardiness skills enhances possibilities for success and leadership for adolescents as they grow into adulthood and may help them during various dilemmas to be faced in life. The results are to be seen in the context of some related research evidence. For example, hardiness is reported to be having a direct effect on self-perceived creativity (61). Also, hardiness is found to be correlated with innovative behavior, the correlation reaching statistical significance in case of challenge component of hardiness only

(62). The results of the study suggest that the existence of hardiness encourages openness to other people and a willingness to strike out in uncharted directions.

School climate has also been found to have significant effect on commitment, challenge and psychological hardiness among adolescents. It has been observed that hardiness significantly affects alienation among student teachers (63). Alienation levels of high-hardy students decreased in more supportive school climate. Indirect relationships for school, gender of the adolescent, hardiness and family coherence has also been found (64). These results are inline with the results of the study which found significant relationship of hardiness with student effort, clinical learning environment and student- faculty relationship among Thai nursing graduates (8). Thus, the findings of the present study pertaining to psychological hardiness vis-à-vis creativity and school climate have a theoretical and empirical support from the literature and these are logical and relevant to explain adolescents' development perspective for future life.

In a rapidly changing world, the cultivation of a creative personality, sensitive and open to problems in his environment, is not only important but is also urgent. A special care and personalized support system is, therefore, imperative to nourish the creative potential of children. Creative talent is expressed in diverse area. As a result of varying areas of talent and individual differences, schools should design unique child-centred educational programmes. There should be environment of psychological freedom, which implies giving the individual complete freedom of symbolic expression, thereby encouraging the spontaneous juggling of ideas, concepts and meaning and psychological safety, to make errors, to bring forth unfinished thought products without being afraid of harsh external evaluation.

Psychological hardiness is conceptualized as a personal stance that facilitates coping effectively with stressful circumstances by accepting them as a natural part of living, and working actively to transform them so that they become less stressful. So, it is suggested that hardiness training should be an important aspect of school enrichment programme Hardiness training has been used effectively with "at risk" students in college and university institutions (65-68). School improvement should be seen as a major focus for all schools, not just those in difficulties. Widening educational opportunities and equity and improving students' attainment levels and social and effective outcomes is essential to promoting active citizens capable and motivated to participate in a democratic society. We need to adopt policies and create schools systems that foster collaboration and create a positive culture for learning with high expectations and recognise that schools do make a difference, that good teaching matters and that we already know much about strategies and practices which foster success for all students.

Like any other research endeavor, the present study has a few limitations. Firstly, the population of the study was delimited to the adolescents studying in eleventh grade in government secondary schools of Punjab state of India. Also, creativity was assessed on the basis of verbal tests of creative thinking only. The secondary school students were classified with high and low levels of creative thinking on the basis of P_{75} and P_{25} cut points to be designated as creative and non-creative. The results might vary if non-verbal creativity or the summation of verbal and non-verbal creativity is taken for the identification of creative adolescents. Lastly, analytic approach to analysis i.e., analysis of variance was used in the analysis of data. In the light of these limitations of the present study, following suggestions for further research may be laid down:

- The present investigation was undertaken on secondary school boys and girls of 10+1 class. This study may be further extended to college and university students and adults.
- The sample of the present investigation included students of the same grade and approximately of the same age. The same may be expanded to cover various age and grade levels in order to make age-wise and grade-wise comparison.
- Only verbal measure of creativity was used to assess the creativity of the subjects. Non-verbal or figural creativity was not assessed. The results may vary if both verbal as well as figural measures are employed. The investigation using both types of measures, need to be designed so as to ascertain if a differential picture of the phenomenon emerges as a consequence of varying impact of both kinds of creative thinking.
- Different school systems are characterized by differential students of excellence in teaching, curricular and co-curricular activities and stimulation for creative and intellectual growth. It will be a useful research endeavor to compare adolescents from different school systems, such as government and private, Navodya and Central, and Public and Ordinary, on the phenomenon studied in this investigation.
- More socio-psychological variables can be incorporated in the research design to determine their possible influence on psychological hardiness.
- Socially disadvantaged group of students may be the focus of some researches to determine socio-psychological correlates of hardiness.
- Experimental studies may be undertaken to determine effect of certain curricular strategies and innovative methods of teaching on hardiness and creativity among school-going adolescents.

REFERENCES

[1] Morrison A, McIntyre D. Schools and socialization. Harmondworth: Penguin Educ, 1973.
[2] Kobasa SC. Stressful life events, personality, and health: An Inquiry into hardiness. J Pers Soc Psychol 1979;37:1-11.
[3] Kobasa SC, Maddi SR, Kahn S. Hardiness and health: A prospective study. J Pers Soc Psychol 1982;42:168-77.
[4] Hannah TE, Morrisey Craig. Correlates of psychological hardiness in Canadian adolescents. J Soc Psychol 1986;1271:339-44.
[5] Dillard NL. Hardiness and academic achievement. Diss Abstr Int 1990; 52: 4121-B.
[6] Cozzi LM. The influence of hardiness, stress, and social support on academic achievement among urban commuter students. Diss Abstr Int 1991;52:2339-B.
[7] McHenry Sandra Dahl. Hardiness and student status as a non-cognitive predictor of academic success and achievement for generic baccalaureate nursing students. Diss Abstr Int 1992;53:4593-B.
[8] Baramee J, Blegen MA. New graduate perception of clinical competence: testing a causal model. Int J Nurs Stud 2003;40:389-99.
[9] Hammond LA. Stress and role satisfaction: The mediating effects of social support, hardiness, coping strategies, and gender in academic multiple role persons. Diss Abstr Int 1987;49:736-A.
[10] Carson DK, Araquistain M, Ide B, Quoss B and Weigel R. Stress, strain, and hardiness as predictors of adaptation in farm and ranch families. J Chinese Fam Stud 1994;3:157-74.
[11] Nathawat SS, Rathore S. Influence of hardiness and social support on well-being in elderly men and women. J Clin Psychol 1996;23:92-101.

[12] Latha E. Type A and hardiness. An analysis of its components. J Psychol Res 2001;45: 50-4.
[13] Nunley BL. Stress, hardiness, and psychological distress of elderly spousal care-givers of persons with dementia. Diss Abstr Int 2002;63:742-B.
[14] McCall J. The development of hardiness in women. Proceedings of the Undergraduate Research Conference, 2005.
[15] Simoni PA. Hardiness as a predictor of burnout in nursing. Diss Abstr Int 1987;49:736-A.
[16] Thomson WC. The contribution of school climate and hardiness to the level of alienation experienced by student teachers. Diss Abstr Int 1993;54:2989-A.
[17] Rush MC, Schoael WA, Barnard, SM. Psychological resiliency in the public sector: "hardiness" and pressure for change. J Vocal Behav 1995;46:17-39.
[18] Judkins, SK. Hardiness, stress and coping strategies among mid-level nurse managers: Implications for continuing higher education. Diss Abstr Int 2002;63:2065-A.
[19] Maddi SR, Khoshaba DM, Persoci M, Lu J, Harvey R, Bleecker F. The personality construct of hardiness. J Res Pers 2002;36:72-85.
[20] Pollock SE. Human responses to chronic illness: Physiologic and psychosocial adaptation. Nurs Res 1986;35:90-5.
[21] Narsavage GL, Weaver TE. Physiologic status, coping, and Hardiness as predictors of outcomes in chronic obstructive pulmonary disease. Nurs Res 1994;43:90-4.
[22] Voyce JA. An investigation of the relationship among attributional styles, hardiness, gender, and depression as predictors of coping with real life events by chemically dependent inpatients. Diss Abstr Int 1996;57:3406-A.
[23] Beasley M, Thompson T, Davidson J. Resilience in response to life stress: The effects of coping style and cognitive hardiness. Pers Individ Diff 2003;34:77-95.
[24] Savage, JS. Social support and Personality Hardiness as mediators of stress in professional women. Diss Abstr Int 1986;48:49-A.
[25] Schiavo AM. The relationship between stress, hardiness, and burnout in College of Education Deans. Diss Abstr Int 1990;51:2227-A.
[26] Thomson WC. The contribution of school climate and hardiness to the level of alienation experienced by student teachers. Diss Abstr Int 1993;54(8):2989-A.
[27] Sharpley CF, Dua JK, Reynolds R, Acosta A. The direct and relative efficacy of cognitive hardiness, a behavior pattern, coping behavior and social support as predictors of stress and ill-health. Scand J Behav Ther 1999;1:15-29.
[28] Roberts GL Personal growth and adjustments. Boston: Holbrook press, 1968.
[29] Barron F, Harrington DM. Creativity, intelligence and personality. Ann Rev Psychol 1981;32:439-76.
[30] Guilford JP. The structure of intellect. Psychol Bull 1956;53:267-93.
[31] Renzulli J. The three ring conception of giftedness: A developmental model for creative productivity. In: Strenberg RJ, Davidson JE, eds. Conceptions of giftedness. New York: Cambridge Univ Press, 1986:53-92.
[32] Gupta AK, Sharma SK. Pupils' creativity in different types of institutional climates: A Study. J Individ Educ 1981;6:27-31.
[33] Jarial GS, Sharma AK. Institutional climate and creativity. ISPT J Res 1982;6:26-30.
[34] Mishra BC. Creativity in students of two types of school. J Psychol Res 1986;30:74-7.
[35] Dhalla Tripti. A psycho-educational profile of creative children. Dissertation. New Delhi: Univ Delhi, 1990.
[36] Pradhan C. Effect of school organizational climate on the creativity, adjustment and academic achievement of secondary school students of Orissa. Dissertation. Utkal: Utkal Univ, 1991.
[37] Raw JS, Marjoribanks K. Family and school correlates of adolescents' creativity, morality, and self concept. Educ Stud 1991;17:183-90.
[38] Singh, YK. Creativity of +1 students in relation to their home environment, risk taking tendency and radical conservative attitude. Dissertation. Patiala: Punjabi Univ, 1995.
[39] Herman Miriam. Adolescents' creativity in relation to separation-individuation and different self-representations. Diss Abstr Int 2001;62:2093-B.

[40] Kumari A, Kumar I, Pandey NK. Effect of academic environment on creativity of children. Asian J Psychol Educ 1988;21:7-11.
[41] Veeraraghwan V. A comparative study of organizational climate, leadership adaptability and teacher effectivness in high, average and low performance schools. New Delhi: Dept Educ, Jawahar Lal Nehru Univ, 1986.
[42] Goodrum AD. Perceived influences on school climate and academic achievement for African-American males in sixth grade: Five case studies. Diss Abstr Int 2000;61:3452-A.
[43] Basantia JM, Mukhopadhyaya D. Effect of environmental factors on achievement: a study on rural school students. Educ Rev 2001;44:1-5.
[44] Natarajan R, Dandapani C. Organizational climate and the academic achievement of pupils in schools. Educ Rev 2003;46:16-9.
[45] Lata S. A Study of Educational Attachment as a Function of School Organizational Climate. Recent Res Educ Psychol 2005;10(3-4):100-3.
[46] Johnson B, Stevens JJ. Student achievement and elementary teachers' perceptions of school climate. Learn Environ Res 2006;9:111-22.
[47] Shrivastava PK, Singh Pi. Academic achievement in different school organisarional climate. Indian J Psychol Educ 2006;37:58-61.
[48] Tracy JF. Perceptions of school climate and self concept: An examination of selected social and emotional factors (Social capital, Self-concept). Diss Abstr Int 2007;67:139-A.
[49] Sharma R. Student morale as a correlate of educational environment in the school. Dissertation. Chandigarh: Panjab University, 1983.
[50] Mistry DH. The quality of school life as a function of organizational climate and pupil control ideology. Dissertation. Surat: South Gujarat Univ, 1985.
[51] Misra G, Tiwari BK. Psychological differentiation in Indian children: Role of ecology, quality of schooling and home environment. Indian Educ Rev 1992;27(1):23-35.
[52] Acosta ES. The relationship between school climate, academic self-concept, and academic achievement. Diss Abstr Int 2001;62:1717-A.
[53] DeRosier ME, Newcity J. Students' perceptions of the school climate Implications for school safety. J Sch Violence 2005; 4:3-19.
[54] Stone S, Han M. Perceived school environments, perceived discrimination, and school performance among children of Mexican immigrants. Child Youth Serv Rev 2005;27:51-66.
[55] Zimmer-Gembeck MJ, Chipuer HM, Hanisch M, Creed PA, McGregor L. Relationships at school and stage-environment fit as resources for adolescent engagement and achievement. J Adolesc 2006;29:911-33.
[56] Raw JS, Marjoribanks K. Family and School Correlates of Adolescents' Creativity, Morality, and Self Concept. Educ Stud 1991;17(2):183-90.
[57] Fernandez P, Venkataraman D. Inter-correlation among creative characteristics and Ego states. Recent Res Educ Psychol 2004;9:45-9.
[58] Mehdi B. Test and Manual for verbal tests of creative thinking. Agra: Natl Psychol Corp, 1973.
[59] Nowack KM. Initial development and validation of a stress and health risk factor instrument. J Health Promot 1990;4:173-80.
[60] Sharma ML. Technical handbook for school organizational climate description questionnaire. Surat: South Gujarat University, 1978.
[61] Chan DW. Self-perceived creativity, family hardiness, and emotional intelligence of Chinese gifted students in Hong Kong. J Sec Gift Educ 2005;16:47-56.
[62] Maddi SR, Harvey RH, Khoshaba DM., Lu John L, Persico M, Brow M. The personality construct of hardiness, III: relationship with repression, innovativeness, authoritarianism, and performance. J Person 2006;74(2):575-97.
[63] Thomson WC, Wendt JC. Contribution of hardiness and school climate to alienation experienced by student teachers. J Educ Res 1995;88:269-74.
[64] Henry CS , Robinson LC, Wilson SM. Adolescent perceptions of their family system, parents' behavior, self esteem, and family life satisfaction in relation to their substance use. J Chinese Adolesc Subst Abuse 2004;13:29-59.

[65] Maddi SR. Hardiness training at Illinois Bell Telephone.:Health promotion and evaluation. Stevens Point, WI: Natl Wellness Inst, 1987.
[66] Rice M. The effect of structured hardiness training intervention program for stress on university women. Diss Abstr Int 1997;58(2): 392-A.
[67] Rowe MM. Hardiness as a stress mediating factor of burnout among healthcare providers. Am J Health Stud 1998;14(1):16-20.
[68] Judkins S, Arris L, Keener E. Program evaluation in graduate nursing education: hardiness as a predictor of success among nursing administration students. J Prof Nurs 2005;21(5):314-21.

In: School, Adolescence and Health Issues
Editors: J. Merrick, A. Tenenbaum and H. A. Omar
ISBN: 978-1-62948-702-1

Chapter 6

PARENTAL EXPECTATIONS ON SCHOOL SEX EDUCATION IN A SUBURBAN COMMUNITY

Esther O Asekun-Olarinmoye**, *BSc(Hons), MD, FWACP, Magbagbeola D Dairo, MBBS, FWACP, Ifeoluwapo O Asekun-Olarinmoye, BSc(Hons), MSc and Wasiu O Adebimpe, MBBS, FWACP

Department of Community Medicine, College of Health Sciences, Faculty of Clinical Sciences, Osun State University, Osogbo, Osun State and Department of Epidemiology and Biostatistics, University College Hospital, Ibadan, Nigeria

ABSTRACT

In this chapter we examined parental expectations on school sex education with 385 parents. A high level of awareness of sex education was found among respondents with a positive attitude towards sex education of their adolescents as two-thirds of respondents affirmed that it should be given to adolescents and four in five parents agreed that sex education should be given in schools. 72.9% want sex education included in the school curriculum and they will support their parents-teachers association (PTA) putting in a request for such although only 16.4% of the respondents had a PTA that had actually requested sex education. 48.8% of the parents would not support free discussion of sex among adolescents in schools. With respect to content of school sex education, majority of the parents want abstinence themes taught while 42.7% want a comprehensive sex education curriculum. Two of five parents (39.5%) did not practice sex education on their children with almost half of the parents reporting that they feel uncomfortable discussing sex issues with their teens. Similarly, majority of the teens (75.8%) do not ask their parents questions about sexual issues. The study concluded that though most parents want their adolescents to have knowledge about sex education, the practice is not well established among these parents because of lack of skill. Community-based sexuality education programmes should be organized for parents to improve their skill. Sex

* Correspondence: Esther Asekun-Olarinmoye, Associate Professor/Clinical Consultant, Department of Community Medicine, College of Health Sciences, Faculty of Clinical Sciences, Osun State University, PMB 4494, Osogbo, Osun State, Nigeria. E-mail: estoaskol@yahoo.com; gmjfunmilayo@gmail.com; estoaskol@uniosun.edu.ng.

education should be introduced into school curriculum with all stakeholders (parents, teachers, government) coming together to fashion out the curriculum contents.

INTRODUCTION

Sex education is a life long process of acquiring information and forming attitudes, beliefs and values. It encourages sexual development, reproductive health, interpersonal relationships, affection, intimacy, body images and gender roles. Sexuality education addresses the biological, socio-cultural, psychological, and spiritual dimension of sexuality from the cognitive domain (information); the affection domain (feelings, values and attitudes); and the behavioral domain (communication and decision making skills). Sexuality education seeks to assist young people in understanding a positive view of sexuality, provide them with information and skills about taking care of their sexual health, and help them make sound decisions now and in the future (1).

Available literature has documented that, in general, adolescents' awareness about sexual and reproductive health issues, for example, certain sexually transmitted infections (STI) is very high; however in-depth knowledge of these issues, which incorporates a deeper understanding of the causes and consequences is low. Thus, many of the consequences of adolescent behavior is almost always due to lack of knowledge about this important issue (2).

Worldwide, adolescents and other young persons (10-24 years) constitute a group at risk of sexually transmitted diseases (STDs) including (Human immunodeficiency Virus) HIV. The risk is indicated in the large proportion of adolescents and other young persons who had unprotected sex with multiple partners (3-6), and in the higher rate at which they become infected with STDs in comparison with older age groups (6,7). The prevalence of HIV/AIDS and STDs within the age group of 15-19 years and 20-24 years is alarming (8). The level of sexual activities and the incidence of STDs are high among Nigerian adolescents, but the use of reproductive health services is low (9).

Debates about sex education have focused on two different approaches: "safe sex" courses, which encourage teens to use contraceptives, especially condoms, when having sex, and "abstinence education", which encourages teens to delay sexual activity. Advocates for Youth have promoted another apparent alternative, entitled "comprehensive sexuality education" or "abstinence plus." These curricula allegedly take a middle position, providing a strong abstinence message while also teaching about contraception (10).

The Alan Guttmacher Research Institute, based on a nationwide survey of school superintendents in the United States of America, found that local policies overwhelmingly encourage abstinence, however public opinion of Americans favor broader sexuality education programs over those that discuss only abstinence (11). Most parents (65%) believe that sex education should encourage young people to delay sexual activity but also prepare them to use birth control and practice safe sex once they do become sexually active. According to interviews conducted for the Kaiser Family Foundation in 2000, majority of respondents said that schools should teach adolescents how to get tested for HIV/AIDS and other STDs (86%), how to talk to a partner about birth control and STDs (77%), how to use condoms (71%), and where to get and how to use other birth control methods (68%) (12).

However, this trend seems to be changing; a poll conducted to assess what parents want taught in sex education programs by Robert et al. in 2004 shows overwhelming parental support for abstinence themes such as "Teenagers should be taught that sex should be linked to marriage; delaying sex until marriage is best, to delay sexual activity until they are married or close to marriage, that abstinence is best, that sex at an early age, sex with many partners, and casual sex have harmful consequences, that the younger the age an individual begins sexual activity, the greater the probability of harm''(10). These are major themes of abstinence programs.

In Nigeria, adolescents face many health risks with too little information, too little guidance about sexual responsibilities and too little access to health care; and except where there has been an intervention, the knowledge of adolescents regarding sexual and reproductive health issues is very poor. There is the likelihood that some of these negative outcomes of adolescent sexual behaviors would be averted where there is adequate knowledge about sexual and reproductive health issues (2). Hence, this study aims to examine parental expectations on school sex education; and what parents want included in the sex education curriculum.

OUR STUDY

This is a descriptive cross-sectional study, conducted in Offatedo, a suburban community, in Osun State, South Western Nigeria. The study population were parents in the community. The sample size calculation assumed that 92.0% of the respondents wanted inclusion of sex education into the school curriculum (13) and anticipated a 20% non-response rate. A minimum sample size of 135 was arrived at using the $n = Z^2pq/d^2$ expression (14). However, a total of 385 parents were selected using cluster random sampling method and they were interviewed using a structured questionnaire. The questionnaire had 4 sections, the socio-demographic characteristics, knowledge and perception about sex education, attitude towards sex education, and practice of sex education. Data extracted from questionnaires were analyzed using Statistical Package for Social Scientists (SPSS) version 15. The results were subjected to appropriate statistical analysis utilizing chi-square test statistics at 95% confidence interval and p-value of <0.05. Approval for the study was obtained from the Ethical Committee of the Department of Community Medicine, Ladoke Akintola University of Technology, Osogbo, and written informed consent was sought and obtained from each respondent.

FINDINGS

A total of 385 parents were interviewed, out of which 45.7% were males (fathers) and 53.2% (mothers) were females. A little above half (55.1%) of the parents interviewed were above the age of 40 years while just 0.5% (2) was below 20 years of age. Majority (91.7%) of our respondents were married, 66.5% in monogamous relationships with 70.4% having adolescents in their homes (Table 1). Two hundred and eighty-six (74.3%) respondents were aware of sex education for adolescents. Sources of information included Radio (55.6%), Newspaper (17.4%), Television (26.8%), friends (19.5%) and relatives (8.8%).

Table 1. Socio-demographic characteristics of respondents

N= 385

Variable	Characteristics	Frequency (n/%)
PARENT	Father	176 (45.7)
	Mother	209 (54.3)
AGE (in years)	Below 20	2 (0.5)
	20-24	12 (3.1)
	25-29	40 (10.4)
	30-34	53 (13.8)
	35-39	66 (17.1)
	40-44	48 (12.5)
	45-49	51 (13.2)
	Above 49	113 (29.4)
MARITAL STATUS	Married	353 (91.7)
	Single	9 (2.3)
	Widow/Widower	12 (3.1)
	No response	11 (2.9)
FAMILY TYPE	Monogamous	256 (66.5)
	Polygamous	103 (26.8)
	No response	26 (6.7)
RELIGION	Christian	196 (50.9)
	Muslims	175 (45.5)
	Traditional	5 (1.3)
	No response	9 (2.3)
ADOLESCENT PRESENT IN THE FAMILY	Yes	271 (70.4)
	No	114 (29.6)

Table 2. Attitude of parents towards sex education

N=385

Attitudinal statements	Agree (n/%)	Disagree (n/%)
Sex education should be given to adolescents	250 (64.9)	135 (35.1)
Sex education should also be given in schools	311 (80.7)	74 (19.3)
Issues relating to sex can be discussed freely among adolescents in schools	197 (51.2)	188 (48.8)
Sex education should be included in school curriculum	281 (72.9)	104 (27.1)
Feel comfortable talking to your children about sex	216 (56.1)	169 (43.9)
PTA requested for inclusion in curriculum	63 (16.4)	322 (83.6)
Support PTA's request	281 (73.0)	104 (27.0)

Table 3. Parental expectations of contents of sex education curriculum for secondary schools

Variables	N=281 Frequency (n/%)
Abstinence until marriage	242 (86.1)
Abstinence until commitment	39 (13.9)
Comprehensive sexuality education	120 (42.7)
Family planning education	68 (24.2)
Use of contraception	46 (16.4)

*Multiple responses.

Table 2 shows the attitude of respondents towards issue on sex education. More than half (64.9%) of our respondents want sex education to be given to adolescents. Majority (80.7%) support that sex education should also be given in school, and 72.9% said sex education should be included in the school curriculum. More than forty percent (43.9%) of parents interviewed said they do not feel comfortable discussing issues of sex with their children.

Of the 281 respondents that wanted sex education to be included in the school curriculum, more than three quarters (86.1%) want abstinence until marriage taught, while just 13.9% want abstinence until commitment to be the content. Furthermore, 42.7% of them wanted comprehensive sex education, and about a quarter (24.2%) wanted the content to include family planning education. (Table 3)

Table 4 shows the distribution of the respondents according to practice of sex education. About two-thirds (60.5%) of parents interviewed said they do give sex education to their children; 21.5% give sex education to their female children only, 3.9%, to their male children only, and 74.8% to both their male and female children. Almost half (47.2%) of the respondents gave sex education occasionally, while about one quarter gave sex education frequently and always respectively. Majority (75.8%) of the respondents' children do not ask their parents questions about sexual issues.

Table 4. Practice of sex education among respondents

Variables	Responses	Frequency (n/%)
Gives sex education to children (n=385)	Yes No	233 (60.5) 152 (39.5)
Gender of children given sex education (n=233)	Females only Males only Both	50 (21.5) 9 (3.9) 174 (74.8)
Frequency of sex education given (n=233)	Always Frequently Occasionally	62 (26.6) 61 (26.2) 110 (47.2)
Children ask parents questions about sex (n=385)	Yes No	93 (24.2) 292 (75.8)
Gender of children that ask parent questions about sex (n=93)	Male Female Both	21 (5.5) 33 (8.8) 39 (14.0)
Comfortable talking to your teen about sex (n=385)	Yes No	216 (56.1) 169 (43.9)

Table 5 shows the distribution of the parents that practiced sex education on their children according to the content being taught. Most of the parents were concerned with the HIV/AIDS epidemic (63.5%) as it was very high on their list of topics taught including other sexually transmitted diseases (57.1%) and puberty changes (52.4%) while issues of most concern that parents discussed with their teens included sexual abstinence (85.8%), the responsibilities of parenthood (69.1%) and abortion and its consequences (67.4%).

Table 5. Content of sexuality education practiced by parents

N= 233

Content	Frequency (%)
TOPICS TAUGHT BY PARENTS IN SEX EDUCATION OF THEIR CHILDREN:	
HIV/AIDS	(63.5)
Deviant sexual behaviour	(56.2)
Sexual reproduction	102 (43.8)
Sexually transmitted diseases	133 (57.1)
Knowledge of contraception	61 (26.2)
Puberty changes	122 (52.4)
Act of Sex	45 (19.3)
SEXUALITY ISSUES DISCUSSED WITH TEENS	
Handling of sexual pressures	(24.9)
Types of birth control	(22.3)
Responsibility of parenthood	161 (69.1)
Sexual abstinence	200 (85.8)
Prostitution	134 (57.5)
Abortion and consequences	157 (67.4)

*Multiple choices.

DISCUSSION

The study found a high level of awareness of sex education among the respondents with about three out of four of them being aware. With adolescents found in majority (70.4%) of the homes studied, the importance of sex education among these adolescents cannot be overemphasized since they constitute at risk group for sexually transmitted diseases (STDs) including Human Immunodeficiency Virus (HIV) (3-7), unwanted pregnancy leading to abortion with its complications (15-17), and other sequelae of risky sexual behaviors (18, 19).

This study found a positive attitude amongst the parents towards sex education of their children as more than half (64.9%) of our respondents wanted sex education to be given to adolescents; majority (80.7%) supported sex education to be given in school, and about three quarters opined that sex education should be included in the school curriculum. However, two of five parents said they do not feel comfortable discussing issues about sex with their children. This finding is in keeping with reports from other researchers from other developing and developed countries (20-22). This lack of ability or skill to discuss issues about sex with their children may be the reason why most parents interviewed in this study wanted sex education to be giving in school (80.7%) or be included in the school curriculum (72.9%). This will thus complement what is given at home by parents who give sex education as well as fill the vacuum for adolescents who do not get sex education from their parents. However, parents should not shift the responsibility of sex education on the teachers because of their own lack of skill. This is an important issue that needs the attention of community-based intervention program planners.

Parental expectations on the content of sex education curriculum in schools consisted mostly of abstinence theme as more than three quarters wanted abstinence until marriage. These abstinence themes programs were also supported by an overwhelming majority of parents in Robert et al.'s study (10). Only two fifth of the respondents wanted the sex education curriculum content to be comprehensive sex education, while just 24.2% wanted family planning education to be included. This differs from Alan Guttmacher Institute research's study on public opinion of Americans in 2001, which favor broader sexuality education programs over those that discuss only abstinence (11), as well as interviews conducted for the Kaiser Family Foundation in 2000 (12). This is probably due to the fact that majority of the parents in this study are not young couples, they belong to the older generation, thus they are expectedly following the normal conservative African traditional culture in regards to sexual issues and child upbringing. This is coupled with most parents' anxiety of preventing STI/HIV infection and unwanted pregnancy with its fatal complications in their adolescents.

Statistics similar to our study was however found in a study conducted by The Heritage Foundation in 2004, where the new poll of parental attitudes shows that less than 10 percent of parents' support the main values and messages of comprehensive sex education programs even in a developed country. Parents overwhelmingly reject main values and messages of comprehensive sex education while they show overwhelming parental support for abstinence themes (10). This shows that parents now prefer abstinence themes to be the major content of sex education curriculum as against comprehensive sex education because comprehensive sex-education curricula are focused almost exclusively on promoting contraceptive use and contain little or no mention of abstinence (10). It thus seems that with the HIV scourge on, most parents will rather have the children taught abstinence rather than use of contraceptive devices.

We conclude that though many parents want their adolescents to have knowledge about sex education, the practice is not well established among these parents. It was also found that most parents want sex education to be included in school curriculum with the contents teaching about abstinence themes. We recommend that parents should be enlightened to encourage them to discuss issues pertaining to sex with their children comfortably. Community-based sexuality education programmes should be organized for parents to improve their skill. Sex education should be introduced into school curriculum with all stakeholders (parents, teachers, government) coming together to fashion out the curriculum contents.

ACKNOWLEDGEMENT

The authors wish to acknowledge the cooperation of parents surveyed in providing necessary information, and the medical students from College of Health Sciences, Ladoke Akintola University of Technology, who were trained as research assistants to help in the data collection.

REFERENCES

[1] The Sex Information and Education Council of the United States (SIECUS). Sexuality education. International Encyclopedia of Marriage and Family, 2003. URL: www. encyclopedia. com/topic/Sex_education.aspx

[2] Action Health Incorporated (AHI). Adolescent sexual and reproductive health in Northern Nigeria: Understanding the contexts and challenges. Lagos, Nigeria: AHI, 2003:43-4,60-2.

[3] Makinwa-Adebusoye PK. Adolescent Reproductive Health Behavior in Nigeria, a study of five cities. NISER monograph series 1990;2:9.

[4] Sonestein FL, Pleck JH, Ku LC. Sexual activities, condom use and AIDS awareness among adolescent males. Fam Plann Perspect 1989; 21:152-58.

[5] Orubuloye OI, Caldwell P, Caldwell JC. The role of high risk occupations in the spread of AIDS: Truck drivers and itinerant market women in Nigeria. Int Fam Plann Perspect 1993;19(2):43-8.

[6] World Health Organization (WHO). School health education to prevent AIDS and sexually transmitted diseases. Geneva: WHO AIDS series, 1989;10:992.

[7] World Health Organization (WHO). Sexually transmitted diseases among adolescents in developing countries. A review of published literature. Geneva: WHO, 1993:10.

[8] McCauley AP, Salter C. Meeting the reproductive health needs of young adults. Population Report Series, John Hopkins University School of Public Health, Baltimore. Population information programme 1995;41: 5. URL: info.k4health.org/pr/j41/j41print.shtml

[9] Temin MJ. Perceptions of sexual behavior and knowledge about sexually transmitted diseases among adolescents in Benin City, Nigeria. Int Fam Plann Perspect 1999;25(4):186-90.

[10] Rector RE, Pardue MG, Martin S. What do parents want taught in sex education programs? Washington, DC: Heritage Foundation 2004;1722:1-21.

[11] Dailard C. Sex education: Politicians, parents, teachers and teen. Guttmacher Report Public Policy 2001;4(1):9-12.

[12] The Henry J Kaiser Family Foundation/ABC Television. Sex in the 90s: 1998 National Survey of Americans on Sex and Sexual Health, Sep 1998.

[13] Orji EO and Esimai OA. Introduction of sex education into Nigerian schools: the parents', teachers', and students' perspectives. J Obstet Gynaecol 2003;23(2):185-8.

[14] Araoye MO. Research methodology with statistics for health and social sciences. Ilorin, Nigeria: Nathadex Publishers, 2003.

[15] WHO. Complications of abortion. URL: www.who.int/entity/.../publications/...abortion/.../index.html

[16] Strahan T. Differential adverse impact of abortion on teenagers who undergo induced abortion. Assoc Interdiscipl Res Bull 2000;15(1):3.

[17] Sobie MR, Reardon DC. The detrimental effects of adolescent abortion. Post-Abortion Rev 2001;9(1):1-5.

[18] Rector RE, Johnson KA, Noyes LR, Martin S. The harmful effects of sexual activity and multiple sexual partners among women: A book of charts. Washington, DC: Heritage Foundation, 2003.

[19] Malhotra S. Impact of sexual revolution: Consequences of risky sexual behavior. J Am Physicians Surgeons 2008;13(3):88-90.

[20] Olakunmi OO, Akintomide AG. Who breaks the ice in parent-child sexual communication-counseling implication for adolescent health and development. Int J Cross-Discipl Subj Educ 2010;1(2):88-92.

[21] Luwaga CNL. Parent-adolescent communication on sexuality in the context of HIV/AIDS in Uganda: an exploratory study. URL: org.uib.no/satz/public/publications/Luwaga%20Master%20Thesis.pdf

[22] Burgess V, Dzieqielewski SF, Green CE. Improving comfort about sex communication between parents and their adolescents: practice-based research within a teen sexuality group. Brief Treat Crisis Intervent 2005;5(4):379-90.

In: School, Adolescence and Health Issues
Editors: J. Merrick, A. Tenenbaum and H. A. Omar
ISBN: 978-1-62948-702-1

Chapter 7

EXPOSURE OF HIGH SCHOOL STUDENTS TO NOISE FROM PERSONAL MUSIC PLAYERS

Benoît Lévesque*, MD, FRCP[1], Raphaëlle Fiset[2], Laurence Isabelle[2], Denis Gauvin, MSc[1], Julie Baril, MPA[3], Richard Larocque, MPA[1], Suzanne Gingras, MSc[1], Tony Leroux, PhD[3], Michel Picard, PhD[3] and Serge André Girard, MA[1]

[1]Institut national de santé publique du Québec, Québec, Canada
[2]École secondaire Les Compagnons de Cartier, Québec, Canada
[3]École d'audiologie de l'Université de Montréal, Montréal, Canada

ABSTRACT

In this chapter we measure noise exposure of students between 14-17 years of age, linked to the use of a personal music player. Specifically, we wanted to estimate the habitual use and sound levels of their music player as well as verify perceptions and habits of youth with regard to recreational noise in relation to their exposure stemming from personal music players. Methods: Students completed a questionnaire on hearing and exposure to recreational noise. We next offered to measure the level of noise exposure from their personal music player. Noise dosimetry in dBA was conducted using the « *Symphonie Program* ». An equivalent 8-hour exposure ($L_{Aeq,8h}$) was measured in relation to exposure from their personal audio players. Variables from the questionnaire were examined in relation with noise exposure using chi-squared tests. Results: Of the 164 students having completed the questionnaire, 141 used a personal music player and of these, 124 agreed to have their player's sound level evaluated. Mean $L_{Aeq,8h}$ from the player was 82.59 dBA, with a range reaching 110.34 dBA. Respective proportions of 60% (75/124) and 42% (52/124) of teenagers were exposed to $L_{Aeq,8h}$ sound levels of 80 dBA and 85 dBA. Conclusion: Youth and their parents must be made aware of the harmful long term effects of noise on hearing and on ways to protect oneself in regard to the use of personal music

* Correspondence: Benoit Lévesque, Institut national de santé publique du Québec, 945, Avenue Wolfe, Québec, Canada, G1V 5B3. Tel : 418-650-5115, ext. 5214; Fax : 418-654-3144; E-mail: Benoit.levesque@ inspq.qc.ca.

players. Governmental authorities worldwide should also consider setting standards concerning the noise levels for personal music players.

INTRODUCTION

Hearing loss due to noise is the most prevalent occupational risk in the world (1) and has led many industrialized countries to implement regulations on occupational noise (1). Exposure to excessive noise is not restricted to the workplace but also include noisy activities. However, such noises, notably stemming from recreational activities, have only been scantily documented to date (1). In the case of recreational activities, teenagers are particularly exposed to noise, including among others, motorised sports, attending concerts, frequenting discotheques and the use of personal music players (1).

The study presented herein is the fruit of a collaboration between two students of a Quebec City high school, the Institut national de santé publique du Québec and the École d'orthophonie et d'audiologie de l'Université de Montréal. It was conducted in view to be presented at the Bell Science Fair 2008 (2), a scientific competition open to high school students from across the province of Quebec. The general objective was to measure the noise exposure of students between 14-17 years of age, linked to the use of a personal music player. Specifically, we aimed at estimating the habitual use and sound levels of their audio player and to verify socio demographic characteristics, perceptions and habits of youth regarding recreational noise in relation to their exposure stemming from personal music players.

OUR STUDY

The population sample was composed of students from l'École secondaire des Compagnons de Cartier, Quebec City, Canada. In total, 196 participants were solicited. The project was approved by the school committee. Parents received a letter explaining the project. Each participant as well as one parent had to sign the consent form of the Bell Science Fair 2008. Data collection was conducted in January and February 2008.

A questionnaire based on tools previously tested by Ahmed et al. (3) and Biassoni et al. (4) was used. The questionnaire primarily consisted of questions on socio-demographics, perception of hearing and on risk due to noise exposure, use of a personal music player and exposure to noise during recreational activities.

For personal music player users, daily listening time during the week and on weekends, as well as the listening level of the player were verified. Noise measurements from the player were conducted using a Type 1 sound level meter whose data was managed by the Symphonie computer program (01 dB-Metravib). This system was adequately calibrated prior to each measurement session. For the measurements, the in-ear earphones were attached to a 2cc coupler representing the size of the external auditory canal of an average adult with this type of device. For on-ear earphones, data was weighted in the laboratory to equal 6 cc, which represents the average volume of the occluded ear of an adult ear. Participants chose their favourite audio piece and adjusted the volume to the level they usually listen to. Participants were then asked to adjust the volume to the maximum level that they would adjust their player. For each of these adjustments, a 2-minute measurement was taken. Sound levels were measured in dBA.

For each participant, the average intensity measured and the daily average length of use after weighting for weekly use (Monday to Friday) and weekend use (Saturday and Sunday) were recorded. The equivalent continuous A-weighted sound for 8 hours ($L_{Aeq,8h}$) was then calculated by the following equation:

$$L_{Aeq,8h} = L_{Aeq,T} + 10 \,\mathrm{Log}_{10} (T/8)$$

where T is time of exposure and $L_{Aeq,T}$ is the equivalent continuous sound measured for time T. This index was used to determine subjects of groups most exposed and groups least exposed on the basis of two different thresholds used as references in the workplace: $L_{Aeq,8h}$ = 80 dBA (5) and $L_{Aeq,8h}$= 85 dBA (6, 7).

The different variables of interest were compared between the groups most and least exposed according to a $L_{Aeq,8h}$ of 80 dBA and a $L_{Aeq,8h}$ of 85 dBA using chi-squared (χ^2) tests. The Mantel Haenszel χ^2 test was also used to verify trends when relevant. Finally, $L_{Aeq,8h}$ means were compared according to type of personal music players (in-ear or on-ear earphones) using the Student's *t* test.

Table 1. Characteristics of participants having completed the questionnaire (n = 164) and personal music player users who participated in the noise study (n = 124)

Variable	Questionnaire		Noise study		
	n*	%	n*	%	P†
Socio-demographics					
Gender					
M	115	70.1	83	66.9	0.56
F	49	29.9	41	33.1	
Age (years)					
14	51	31.1	40	32.3	0.95
15	59	36.0	41	33.1	
16	45	27.4	35	28.2	
17	9	5.5	8	6.4	
Education					
High school III	63	38.4	47	37.9	0.43
High school IV	62	37.8	45	36.3	
High school V	39	23.8	32	25.8	
Hearing perception					
Tinnitus					
Yes	23	14.0	14	11.3	0.49
No	141	86.0	110	88.7	
Tinnitus after listening to audio input					
Yes	9	5.5	5	4.0	0.56
No	154	94.5	119	96.0	
Television volume at a higher level than previous year					
Yes	36	22.0	26	21.0	0.84
No	128	78.0	98	79.0	

Table 1. (Continued)

Variable	Questionnaire		Noise study		P†
	n*	%	n*	%	
Hearing compared to 5 years ago					
Better	9	5.5	7	5.7	0.88
Unchanged	129	78.7	100	80.6	
Worse	26	15.8	17	13.7	
Hearing compared to a person of the same age					
Better	31	18.9	24	19.4	0.98
Same	105	64.0	80	64.5	
Worse	28	17.1	20	16.1	
Use of personal music player					
Use of a player					
Yes	141	87.0	124	100	<0.001
No	21	13.0	0	0	
Since when					
< 1 year	15	10.6	12	10.2	0.98
1-2 years	40	28.4	32	27.1	
3-5 years	67	47.5	59	50.0	
> 5 years	19	13.5	15	12.7	
Number of hours used compared to the previous year					
Same	60	47.6	52	49.1	0.97
+	36	28.6	30	28.3	
-	30	23.8	24	22.6	
Type of listening device					
In-ear	110	82.7	98	79.0	0.45
On-ear	23	17.3	26	21.0	
Perception of volume too high					
Subject					
Never	21	14.9	14	11.9	0.90
Occasionally	101	71.6	88	74.6	
Often	16	11.3	14	11.9	
Always	3	2.1	2	1.6	
Entourage					
Never	71	50.4	56	47.5	0.95
Occasionally	54	38.3	48	40.7	
Often	13	9.2	12	10.2	
Always	3	2.1	2	1.7	
Risk perception of excessive noise from audio					
Yes	153	93.3	115	92.7	0.86
No	11	6.7	9	7.3	
Noisy recreational activities					
Noisy activities in the last year					
Yes	63	38.4	46	37.1	0.82
No	101	61.6	78	62.9	
Playing of a musical instrument					
Yes	60	36.6	47	37.9	0.82
No	104	63.4	77	62.1	

* For certain variables, numbers are lower due to non-respondents.

† p value calculated by χ^2 test.

Table 2. Listening habits of participants who had their personal music player evaluated (n=124)

	Mean	Standard deviation	Range
Listening time/day (hours)			
Week	1.55	1.06	0.17 – 5.00
Weekend	1.01	1.09	0 – 5.50
$L_{Aeq,8h}$* (dBA)	82.59	11.89	51.45 – 110.34
$L_{Aeq,2min\ mean}$† (dBA)	91.13	10.82	62.40 – 113.20
$L_{Aeq,2\ min\ max}$‡ (dBA)	99.23	10.71	69.40 - 122.30

* Equivalent continuous sound for 8 hours.

† Mean equivalent continuous sound for 2 minutes.

‡ Maximum equivalent continuous sound for 2 minutes.

FINDINGS

Of the 196 students invited to complete the online questionnaire, 164 (84%) participated in the study. Of this group, 141 (86%) used a personal music player of which 124 (88%) agreed to allow us evaluate their exposure to noise from their player. Table 1 presents the characteristics of study participants. Aside from the fact that all participants had to be users of a personal music player, there was no significant difference ($p > 0.4$) for the main variables between the group of respondents to the questionnaire and the sub-group who participated in the study on noise. Globally, participants were predominantly boys distributed almost evenly across the different age groups.

Table 2 presents the listening habits of participants. Overall, 60% (75/124) and 42% (52/124) of the students were exposed to noise levels over a $L_{Aeq,8h}$ of 80 dBA and 85 dBA respectively. With regard to the type of listening devices, there was no significant difference ($p = 0.19$) between means of $L_{Aeq,8h}$ for on-ear devices ($L_{Aeq,8h}$, mean= 79.86, S.D. = 10.12) and in-ear devices ($L_{Aeq,8h}$, mean= 83.32, S.D. = 11.58).

Tables 3 and 4 present a comparative analysis of variables of interest between users of personal music players as a function of $L_{Aeq,8h}$ noise levels of 80 dBA and 85 dBA respectively.

DISCUSSION

A proportion of 87% of participating students used a personal music player, of which approximately 50% have been using this type of audio device for a period of 3 to 5 years (see table 1). The observed mean listening time of over 1-hour per day of use (see table 2) confirms that personal music players are indeed omnipresent in the daily life of participating youth. Moreover, the characteristics of those having completed the questionnaire were not different from the sub-group who subsequently participated in the noise study. These data are reassuring as to the generalisation of results to the overall respondents to the questionnaire.

However, the school where the study was conducted was ranked in the first decile of the socio-economic index of the Ministère de l'Éducation, du Loisir et du Sport du Québec (8) in 2007-2008, therefore serving a well-to-do clientele, which may not be entirely representative of the reality of youth from more disadvantaged backgrounds.

Table 3. Comparison of variables of interest between adolescents stratified according to an equivalent continuous A-weighted sound of more than 80 dBA for 8 h

Variable	≤ 80		> 80		p*
	n	%	n	%	
Gender					
F	16	32.6	25	33.3	0.93
M	33	67.4	50	67.7	
Age					0.05†
14	13	26.5	27	36.0	0.07
15	13	26.5	28	37.3	
16-17	23	46.9	20	26.7	
Education					0.02†
High school III	14	28.6	33	44.0	0.06
High school IV	17	34.7	28	37.3	
High school V	18	36.7	14	18.7	
Tinnitus					
Yes	2	4.1	12	16.0	0.04
No	47	95.9	63	84.0	
Listening volume					
< ½	21	42.9	13	17.3	0.001
½ - ¾	28	57.1	53	70.7	
> ¾	0	0	9	12.0	
Perception of volume too high					
Subject					
Never/Occasionally	46	100	56	77.8	0.0006
Often/Always	0	0	16	22.2	
Entourage					
Never/Occasionally	42	91.3	62	86.1	0.39
Often/Always	4	8.7	10	13.9	
Noisy activities in the previous year					
Yes	12	24.5	35	46.7	0.01
No	37	75.5	40	53.3	

* p value calculated by χ^2 test.

† p value calculated by the Mantel-Haenszel χ^2 test.

More than 20% of participants estimated having increased the volume of the television over the past year and approximately 15% judged their hearing to be worse than 5 years ago (see table 1). Admittedly, it is difficult to interpret such perceptions which may be the object of bias and further compounded by that fact that participants were made aware of the effects of noise on hearing through their science program at school. Furthermore, more than 10% of participants mentioned having tinnitus in general and approximately 5% after listening to their music player (see table 1). Documenting tinnitus is not easy and the question used in the questionnaire was somewhat ambiguous. Nonetheless, a recent study conducted on a sample of over 2,700 Swedish youth aged between 15-16 years showed the prevalence of tinnitus occurring occasionally or rarely, at respectively 9.3% and 19.5% (9). Even when taking into consideration the variations in questionnaires used, these latter numbers documented in a population of the same age are comparable to those in our study. However, our data indicate that the occurrence of tinnitus appears to be as much related to the noise level emanating from the personal music player according to a $L_{Aeq,8h}$ of more than 80 dBA (see table 3) than above 85 dBA (see table 4). Theoretically, such a symptom may represent a premature effect of the use of personal music players on the auditory system.

Table 4. Comparison of variables of interest between adolescents stratified according to an equivalent continuous A-weighted sound of more than 85 dBA for 8 h

Variable	≤ 85		> 85		p*
	n	%	n	%	
Gender					
F	22	30.6	19	36.5	0.48
M	50	69.4	33	63.5	
Age					0.04†
14	19	26.4	21	40.4	0.11
15	23	31.9	18	34.6	
16-17	30	41.6	13	25.0	
Education					0.04†
High school III	22	30.6	25	48.1	0.12
High school IV	28	38.9	17	32.7	
High school V	22	30.6	10	19.2	
Tinnitus					
Yes	5	6.9	9	17.3	0.07
No	67	93.1	43	82.7	
Listening volume					
< ½	27	37.5	7	13.5	0.0006
½ - ¾	44	61.1	37	71.1	
> ¾	1	1.4	8	15.4	
Perception of volume too high					
Subject					
Never/Occasionally	65	94.2	37	75.5	0.003
Often/Always	4	5.8	12	24.5	
Entourage					
Never/Occasionally	64	92.7	40	81.6	0.07
Often/Always	5	7.3	9	18.4	
Noisy activities in the previous year					
Yes	22	30.6	25	48.1	0.05
No	50	69.4	27	51.9	

* p value calculated by χ^2 test.

† p value calculated by the Mantel-Haenszel χ^2 test.

On average, the $L_{Aeq,8h}$ was 82.59 dBA, with the range extending to 110.34 dBA (see table 2). This level was higher (83.32 dBA) in users of in-ear earphones as opposed to on-ear earphones, although the difference was not statistically significant (p= 0.19). Hodgetts et al. (10) in a study among 38 subjects, showed that participants using both types of earphones were less exposed to noise with on-ear devices. Fligor and Cox (11) also concluded that in-ear devices were more inclined to generate a greater exposure to noise. In the present study, approximately 80% of adolescents used in-ear devices (see table 1).

Globally, 60% of participants (75/124) (see table 3) listened to their music player at a level exceeding the European occupational health standards of 80 dBA (8 hours/day, 40 hours/week) (5). Moreover, a further 52 subjects (42 %) (see table 4) were even exposed to a noise intensity equivalent to a $L_{Aeq,8h}$ superior to 85 dBA, the exposure norm generally in force in the workplace (6, 7). This latter threshold was elaborated following studies in the workplace showing the harmful effects of noise on hearing health while estimating the dose-effect relationship (12, 13). While there is no actual scientific evidence allowing us to affirm that noise outside the workplace is a different aggressor with regard to its effects on hearing (5), a 42% prevalence of exposure to a music player equivalent to a $L_{Aeq,8h}$ over 85 dBA (see table 4) is obviously not negligible. All the more so since many participants mentioned being regularly exposed to other noisy activities (discotheques, motorized vehicles, occupational noise…) in the past year, and that exposure to noisy environments was significantly more important in those who were more exposed to noise from their music players (see tables 3 and 4).

Over the years, a small number of studies have documented sound levels generated by personal music players in relation to a $L_{Aeq,8h}$ over 85 dBA, particularly in young adults (3, 14-16). While results were found to vary, they nevertheless showed proportions reaching 25 to 30% (14, 16) of individuals using their player over this limit, that is to say slightly lower than that documented in our study (42%) in subjects generally younger. In this regard, our data show that exposure to noise from a personal music player seems to decrease significantly with age (see table 3, p=0.05; Table 4, p=0.04).

There was also a relationship between the perception of volume being too high by participants and noise dose levels (see tables 3 and 4). It appears difficult for an observer to judge the intensity of the noise of a player as close as 250 cm (7). This possibly explains why only 18% of parents of participants exposed to a $L_{Aeq,8h}$ of 85 dBA and higher were aware of the sound level, even though we did notice a trend (p= 0.07) in the entourage of these youth toward warning them more frequently (see table 4). Despite this fact, these numbers indicate that parents as much as youth should be made aware of the problem. Vogel et al. (17) recently estimated that interventions should be developed to increase knowledge of our youth on the risks linked to personal music players. Our data indicate that parents should also be targeted by such interventions.

The present study shows that efforts must be made to raise both youth and parent awareness relative to the harmful effects of noise from personal music players on hearing and on means to protect users against these ill effects. Following the example of France where the number of decibels is limited to 100 dB (7), and the recent European Commission recommendations to set default volume settings to safe exposure levels (80 dBA for an exposure of 40 hours/week to 89 dBA for an exposure of 5 hours/week) (18) with reliable means to inform users of the risks if they select a deliberately higher level, governmental authorities worldwide should also consider setting standards concerning noise levels for personal music players.

ACKNOWLEDGEMENTS

The authors would like to thank Marie Audet and Sébastien Simard, both teachers at the high school Les Compagnons de Cartier, for their contribution without which this study could not have been conducted. We would also like to thank Susie Bernier, Marie-Christine Gervais, Claire Laliberté, Mélanie Tessier, Étienne Angers and Pierre Pothier. Finally, sincere thanks to the high school students of Les Compagnons de Cartier who agreed to participate in this study.

REFERENCES

[1] World Health Organization. Guidelines for community noise. Geneva: WHO, 1999.

[2] Fiset R, Isabelle L. À s'en péter les tympans. Présentation des projets- Super Expo-Sciences Bell, finale québécoise 2008, #49. URL: http://www.exposciencesbell.qc.ca/fr/pdf/SESB_2008-resume-projets-110408.pdf.

[3] Ahmed S, Fallah S, Garrido B, Gross A, King M, Morrish T, et al. Use of portable audio devices by university students. Can Acoustics 2007;35(1):35-52.

[4] Biassoni EC, Serra MR, Richter U, Joekes S, Yacci MR, Carignani JA, et al. Recreational noise exposure and its effects on the hearing of adolescents. Part II: Development of hearing disorders. Int J Audiol 2005;44(2):74-85.

[5] Scientific Committee on Emerging and Newly Identified Health Risks (SCENIHR). Potential health risks of exposure to noise from personal audio players and mobile phones including a audio playing function. Brussels: Directorate-General for Health and Consumers; European Commission, 2008.

[6] National Institute for Occupational Safety and Health (NIOSH) (1998). Criteria for a recommended standard: Occupational noise exposure, 1998. URL: http://www.cdc.gov/niosh/docs/98-126/

[7] Keith SE, Michaud DS, Chiu V. Evaluating the maximum playback sound levels from portable digital audio players. J Acoust Soc Am 2008;123(6):4227-37.

[8] Ministère de l'Éducation, du Loisir et du Sport du Québec (MELS), 2008. Indices de défavorisation. URL: http://www.mels.gouv.qc.ca/stat/indice_defav/index_ind_def.htm.

[9] Brunnberg E., Linden-Bostrom M., Berglund M. Tinnitus and hearing loss in 15-16 year-old students: mental health symptoms, substance use, and exposure in schools. Int J Audiol 2008;47(11):688-94.

[10] Hodgetts WE, Rieger JM, Szarko RA. The effects of listening environment and earphone style on preferred listening levels of normal hearing adults using an MP3 player. Ear Hear 2007;28(3):290-7.

[11] Fligor BJ, Cox LC. Output levels of commercially available portable compact disc players and the potential risk to hearing. Ear Hear 2004;25(6):513-27.

[12] Burns W, Robinson DW. Hearing and noise in industry. London: HMSO, 1970.

[13] ISO 1999: 1990 Acoustics. Determination of occupational noise exposure and estimation of noise-induced hearing impairment. Geneva: Int Comm Standardisation, 1990.

[14] Catalano PJ, Levin SM. Noise-induced hearing loss and portable radios with earphones. Int J Audiol 1985;9(1):59-67.

[15] Wong TW, Hasselt CAV, Tang LS, Yiu PC. The use of personal cassette players among youths and its effects on hearing. Public Health 1990;104(5):327-30.

[16] Williams W (2005). Noise exposure levels from personal stereo use. Int J Audiol 2005;44(4):231-6.

[17] Vogel I, Brug J, Hosli EJ, van der Ploeg CPB, Raat H. MP3 players and hearing loss: adolescents' perceptions of loud audio and hearing conservation. J Pediat 2008; 152(3):400-4.

[18] Shilov A. European Commission to set default volume settings on personal music players, 2009. URL: http://www.xbitlabs.com/news/multimedia/display/ 20090928085946_European_Commission_to_Set_Default_Volume_Settings_on_ Personal_Music_Players.html

In: School, Adolescence and Health Issues
Editors: J. Merrick, A. Tenenbaum and H. A. Omar
ISBN: 978-1-62948-702-1

Chapter 8

TEENS TEXTING

Archana Srinivas, MD, Megan White, MD and Hatim A Omar, MD*

Division of Adolescent Medicine, Department of Pediatrics, University of Kentucky, Lexington, Kentucky, US

ABSTRACT

In this chapter we summarize the current literature on texting use amongst adolescents. A brief overview will be presented on the prevalence of texting among teenagers, the use of texting for sexting and cyberbullying as well as the dangers of texting while driving. This chapter will serve as a brief overview of these topics in order to bring to light the emerging challenges that texting presents to the mental and physical well-being of adolescents in an effort to evoke further discussion regarding the need for increasing awareness and education to parents, educators, law makers and health care providers concerning these issues.

INTRODUCTION

Since the advent of mobile cellular phones, they have become a staple in everyday life. Although initially intended primarily for making phone calls, today cellular phones are used for a variety of additional purposes including text messaging, social networking, and the exchange of photos and videos. While phone calls still remain the primary use of the cellular phone, text messaging has become the second most common use of the cellular phone (1). According to the Cellular Telecommunications Industry Association (CTIA), in December 2009 alone, an average of 534 text messages was sent per subscriber per month. At first glance, this figure may seem large, until it is compared to the astounding average of 3,339 texts sent per month by teenagers aged 14-17 years (2). In 2010, the Nielsen Company

* Correspondence: Professor Hatim A Omar, MD, FAAP, Director of Adolescent Medicine and Young Parent programs, J422 Kentucky Clinic, Department of Pediatrics, Kentucky Children's Hospital, University of Kentucky College of Medicine, Lexington, KY 40536 United States. E-mail: haomar2@uky.edu.

calculated that female teenagers send 4,050 texts per month and male teenagers send 2,539—figures that have been steadily increasing (2). As with most advancements in technology, young people are the quickest to integrate any new innovations into their personal lives. Text messaging is no exception. It is an extremely popular form of communication that can easily be misused, especially by adolescents with under-developed decision-making capabilities. In this article we will summarize the existing data on three major areas of concern with regard to adolescent texting including: sexting, texting while driving, and cyberbullying.

SEXTING

In recent years, parents, educators, advocates, and the media have become increasingly concerned about the role of cellular phones in adolescent sexual interactions and exploration (3-5). The leading concern is regarding "sexting" a term blended from the words "sex" and "text," that describes sending sexually explicit text messages and images. To determine how widespread this practice is, multiple national surveys have been conducted. One such study, entitled Sex and Tech surveyed teenagers, aged 14-19 years and young adults, age 20-26 years, about the use of cellular phones in their sex lives during the fall of 2008 (3). Thirty-nine percent of surveyed teenagers admitted to sending or posting sexually suggestive messages by text message, email, or instant message, and 28% of teenagers had received such messages (3). One in five teenagers admitted to sending or posting nude or seminude pictures or videos of themselves (3). Interestingly, 44% of teenage girls and 36% of teenage boys believed it was common and possibly even acceptable for these messages to be shared with people other than the recipients (3). Male and female teenagers reported that the main reason to send a message with such content was that it is "fun or flirtatious," (3). With this kind of motive in mind, it is clear that this carefree generation of adolescents may not have a clear understanding of the potential consequences of sexting.

The most troublesome dilemma to this new phenomenon is that it involves including minors in sexually explicit material. Lawmakers and prosecutors have begun to approach this issue around the nation with varying degrees of severity (4). Likewise, teenagers and others are unfortunately discovering that taking images of anyone under the age of 18 years, even if it is oneself, is a state and federal offense (4). In some states, teenagers who have created and distributed such images have been charged under laws that originally were only reserved for those involved with child pornography (4). In Florida, one case labeled an 18-year-old male as a registered sexual offender for 25 years after he distributed nude images of his 16-year-old girlfriend following a quarrel between them (5). This case demonstrates the grave and lasting consequences teenagers may unknowingly face when engaging in the increasingly trendy activity of sexting.

With this rapid increase of teenage sexting, it is essential that parents, educators, even health professionals become vigilant about monitoring the activities of their adolescent children, students, and patients, respectively. Furthermore, it is important to increase awareness regarding the consequences of sexting. By targeting teenagers in multiple settings including school, the healthcare environment and the media can serve to increase awareness regarding the legal and numerous social implications for sexual messaging (6-8).

DRIVING AND TEXTING

The United States Department of Transportation divides distracted driving into three main categories: visual, manual, and cognitive, all of which many drivers do routinely while driving (9). A visual distraction results from the driver taking his eyes off the road. A manual distraction is when the driver removes his hands from the steering wheel, and a cognitive distraction is when the driver is focused on something other than driving (9). In 2009 alone, 20% of injury crashes reported at least one type of distracted driving. While every type of distraction may endanger a driver, the most concerning distracting activity cited is texting while driving due to the fact that it encompasses all three classes of distraction (9). Given the novelty of texting, there are limited statistics regarding the harmful effects of texting while driving; however, there are numerous studies examining the dangers of any cellular phone activity while driving. According to the National Highway Traffic Safety Administration (NHTSA), 18% of fatalities in distraction related cases were related to cellular phone use (9). The age group with the highest incidence of distractions while driving was for people under age 20, where 16% of those involved in a fatal crash reported distractions while driving (9).

Currently, twelve states have banned talking on a cellular phone while driving (9). This measure has encouraged more drivers to actively pursue hands-free alternatives. However, despite the restriction in these states, texting while driving remains a common distraction. In an effort to decrease the distraction of texting, thirty states, the District of Columbia, and Guam have enforced texting restrictions while driving (8). In these states, 12% of drivers reported texting while driving, whereas in states without restrictions, 14% of drivers reported texting while driving (10). Unsurprisingly, drivers aged 18-24 were the most likely offenders including, 45% in texting restricted states, and 48% in unrestricted states (10). This 2010 study revealed that restricting the use of text messaging while driving is unfortunately ineffective in any age group (10). In a similar study focusing on high school students, 45% of teenagers admitted to some sort of cellular phone during their most recent car ride (11). Fifteen percent admitted to only talking on a cellular phone, 15% admitted to sending or reading messages only, and another 15% admitted to talking and texting (11). Astonishingly, these teenagers also reported employing strategies to decrease associated risks while driving. Of those reporting texting and driving, 58% waited until they believed it was safe to read a text message, and 47% to reply to text messages (11).

Recently, a survey of young drivers regarding their perception of the risk of texting and driving revealed conflicting results (12). While drivers admitted that texting while driving was a much riskier behavior than only talking on a cellular phone while driving, this identified risk did not change their choice to participate in texting (12). Interestingly, when drivers perceived safer road conditions according to their own standards, then they more frequently engaged in texting (12). These results are alarming considering that it is apparent that teenagers are able to identify the risk, but are not able to modify their behavior accordingly. Atchlet et al. concluded that engaging in texting behavior decreases the perceived risk of such behavior (12).

In response to the growing concern of texting and driving, many cellular phone providers have since begun to target those most likely to engage in this risky behavior. Verizon wireless began its national "Don't text and Drive" campaign in 2009 while cellular phone giant AT&T started their "Texting & Driving... It can Wait" campaign in 2010 (5, 13). With short videos featuring families with lost loved ones, as well as focus groups, the theme of AT&T's campaign is one that appears to resonate with adolescents: "no text is worth dying over," (13). As with sexting, publicizing the dangers of texting while driving remains an important and effective tool available to promote awareness of the consequences of texting and driving. In the future, new innovative interventions should target adolescents, the most common offenders of texting while driving, to help decrease the injuries and fatalities that are associated with such distracted driving.

Bullying and Texting

The traditional definition of bullying is "an aggressive intentional act or behavior carried out by a group or an individual repeatedly and over time against a victim who cannot easily defend him or herself" (14). With widespread use of technologies in daily activity as described above, it is not surprising that there are new and innovative ways to bully as well. "Cyberbullying" is a recent term used to describe a form of bullying where victims are harassed with electronic forms of contact (15). This new form of bullying became so quickly popularized amongst adolescents that many adults are still unaware of its existence. One online resource that compiles much of the cyberbullying literature into palatable information for adolescents, adults, and educators is the Cyberbullying Research Center (15). The Cyberbullying Research Center estimates that the prevalence of adolescents affected by cyberbullying may range from 10-40%. A study randomly selected 11-18 year old students in 2010 showed that about 20% of these students are victims of cyberbullying (15). An additional 10% admitted to being both a victim and an offender (15).

It is not surprising that cyberbullying results in emotional distress. Recent research shows that there is a dramatic difference regarding the impact cyberbullying may have when compared to traditional face-to-face bullying (15). According to the Cyberbullying Research Center, there are many major differences to address (15). First, victims may be harassed by an anonymous bully, and may not fully understand why they are being targeted (15). Second, with the easy dissemination of information on the Internet, a bullying incident can quickly and easily become public knowledge and a large number of people can become aware of the incident within the push of a few buttons (15). Third, cyberbullying can be easily initiated from a distance, where the bully maybe unaware of the complete effect on their victim and does not have to face the consequences of their actions (15). Additionally, victims never have respite from their cyberbully, as the Internet is available at all hours of the day, not just during school hours (15). Lastly, there are limited consequences to cyberbullying from the majority of adults, who are largely unaware of cyberbullying and how devastating it can be for adolescents (15).

The effects of cyberbullying are similar to those caused by traditional bullying including anxiety, low self esteem, and even suicidal ideation (15). While all forms of bullying result in a greater incidence of suicidal thoughts, victims of cyberbullying were almost twice as likely to have attempted suicide compared to those who had no experience with cyberbullying (15). In 2010 cyberbullying was brought to national attention when there were several teenage suicides thought to be largely influenced by electronic bullying (16-19).

In the future, schools and parents should continue to patrol cellular phone use, as well as Internet access. With schools keeping a diligent no cellular phone use on campus, and parents keeping track of their child's social media activity at home, some instances of cyberbullying may potentially be averted. Additionally, as with sexting and texting while driving, increasing awareness about cyberbullying is crucial to decreasing the incidents and far-reaching consequences of cyberbullying on adolescents.

CONCLUSION

With the exponentially increasing usage of cellular and Internet communication, new dangers that affect teenagers have arisen including sexting, texting while driving, and cyberbullying. As described above, each activity poses a specific hazard to the emotional well-being and physical safety to teenagers. Given these new challenges, it is important to increase the education and awareness about the potentially devastating consequences of sexting, texting while driving, and cyberbullying to the mainstream public, to parents, to educators, and to healthcare professionals. By these efforts, it would be possible to decrease the sexual exploitation of teenagers through sexting, the injuries and fatalities associated with texting and driving, and the anxiety, low self-esteem, and suicidal ideation, associated with cyberbullying, and improve the overall well-being of adolescents in this technologically advancing era.

REFERENCES

[1] CITA Wireless Quick Facts. URL: http://www.ctia.org/consumer_info/ service/ index.cfm/AID/10323.

[2] The Nielsen Company. U. S. Teen Mobile Report: Calling yesterday, texting today, using apps tomorrow. Nielsen Wire 2010. URL: http://blog/nielsen.com/nielsenwire/online_mobile/u-s-teen-mobile-report-calling-yesterday-texting-today-using-apps-tomorrow/.

[3] The National Campaign to Prevent Teen and Unplanned Pregnancy. Sex and tech. URL: http://www.thenationalcampaign.org/sextech/PDF/SexTech_Summary.pdf.

[4] Humbach, J. "Sexting" and the First Amendment 2010. URL: http://digitalcommons. pace.edu/cgi/viewcontent.cgi?article=1594&context=lawfaculty&sei-redir=1#search="sexting".

[5] Feyerick, D and Steffen, S.. "Sexting lands teen on sex offender list" 2009. URL: http://www.cnn.com/2009/CRIME/04/07/sexting.busts/index.html.

[6] Norris, ML. HEADSS up: Adolescents and the Internet. J Paediatr Child Health, 2007: 12(3), 211-6.

[7] Katzman, DK. Sexting: Keeping teens safe and responsible in a technologically savvy world. Paediatr Child Health 2010:15(1):41-2.

[8] American Academy of Pediatrics. Talking to kids and teens about social media and sexting 2011. Accessed 18 Mar 2011. URL: http://www.aap.org/advocacy/releases/june09socialmedia.htm.

[9] Distraction.gov. Statistics and facts about distracted driving. Accessed 22 Mar 2011. URL: http://www.distraction.gov/stats-and-facts/.

[10] Braitman, K and McCartt, A. National reported patterns of driver cell phone use in the United States. Traff Inj Prev 2010:11(6):543-8.

[11] O'Brien N, Goodwin A, Foss R. Talking and texting among teenage drivers: a glass half empty or half full? Traff Inj Prev 2010:11(6): 549-54.

[12] Atchley P, Atwood S, Boulton A. The choice to text and drive in younger drivers: behavior may shape attitude. Acc Anal Prev 2011: 43(1):143-42.

[13] AT&T. It Can Wait Pledge. URL: http://itcanwait.att.com/.
[14] Olweus, D. Bullying at school: what we know and what we can do. Oxford: Blackwell, 1993.
[15] Cyberbullying Research Center. URL:www.cyberbullying.us.
[16] ABC News. Mean girls: Cyberbullying blamed for teen suicides 2010. URL: http://abcnews.go.com/GMA/Parenting/girls-teen-suicide-calls-attention-cyberbullying/story?id=9685026.
[17] Fox News. Rutgers student suicide renews debate over cyberbullying 2010. URL: http://www.foxnews.com/politics/2010/10/01/rutgers-student-suicide-renews-debate-cyberbullying/.
[18] CBS News. Cyberbullying continued after teens death 2010. URL: http://www.cbsnews.com/stories/2010/03/29/earlyshow/main6343077.shtml.
[19] ABC News. Teens indicated after allegedly taunting girl who hanged herself 2010. URL:http://abcnews.go.com/Technology/TheLaw/teens-charged-bullying-mass-girl-kill/story?id=10231357.

In: School, Adolescence and Health Issues
Editors: J. Merrick, A. Tenenbaum and H. A. Omar
ISBN: 978-1-62948-702-1

Chapter 9

SNEAKING AROUND THE STREETS: PROLIFIC GRAFFITI TAGGERS' SOCIALIZATION HABITS

Myra F Taylor, PhD, MPhil, Dip SocSc, BGS*
School of Psychology and Social Science,
Edith Cowan University Western Australia, Australia

ABSTRACT

Tagging, the unsolicited rendition of a graffiti writer's street name on someone else's property is typically committed by adolescents aged 12-17 years who are seeking a deviant non-conforming social identity. While graffiti involvement places prolific writers on a trajectory towards more serious criminal offending, little is known about their tagging practices. To address this knowledge shortfall, an examination was conducted of 1,462 graffiti report forms completed by removalists prior to their removing graffiti written on the city streets of Perth, Western Australia over a three month period. Frequency distribution analysis revealed that while 759 individuals collectively wrote 2,729 tags, just 16 prolific taggers accounted for approximately half (n=1,373) of all the tags recorded. Moreover, a tag frequency tally revealed that while some prolifically written tags appeared in isolation, others occurred in conjunction with a particular set of other tags. Finally, by plotting the occurrences of the 16 identified prolifically written tags on square grid plots, the results demonstrate the existence of graffiti hangout hubs. These findings are discussed in relation to the thesis of Reputation Enhancement and the social non-conforming identity seeking aspirations of adolescent graffiti taggers.

* Correspondence: Myra Taylor, PhD, Research Fellow, School of Psychology and Social Science, Edith Cowan University, WA 6027, Australia. E-mail: myraftaylor@gmail.com.

INTRODUCTION

Sometime between the ages of 12-17 years adolescents typically reach a period of 'identity crisis' during which they not only question the standards imposed on them by adults central to their daily lives, but also actively 'seek out social values and ideologies with which they can identify' (1). Peer affirmation is crucial to this identification process (2). In order to attain peer affirmation adolescents, particularly those in their early teens, tend to suppress the 'non-cool' aspects of their burgeoning-self in order to acquiesce to the collective identity of their mainstream peer-group and smaller friendship cliques (3).

Such groups/cliques normally are differentiated by aspects of clothing, accessories, speech, mannerisms, body markings/piercings, leisure pursuits or hang-out locations. Whereas most juveniles conform to the mores and social norms of their mainstream peer-group and friendship cliques in order to attain their desired social identity, the ensuing process of suppressing self, which inclusion often necessitates, is generally only a transitional period in adolescent social development (4). Thus, by the time adolescents enter adulthood their personal identity is developed to such an extent that they are able to disregard their former peer-group/friendship clique's conformity pressures. Thus, the early-late teen years is an important stage in adolescent social development given it is during this time that adolescents actively seek social acceptance by manifesting behaviours consistent with those of their desired peer-group/clique (5-7). In most typically developing adolescents such manifested behaviours are generally compatible with their desired peer-group/clique's social identity and, hence, inclusion occurs (2).

In a comparatively small number of cases, however, some adolescents fail to secure mainstream peer-group/clique affirmation of their identity seeking actions. As a consequence, these un-affirmed teens tend to either disassociate themselves or are ousted from their mainstream peer-group (8). Once marginalized, self-disassociating or peer-ousted adolescents tend to manifest a range of social-assimilation difficulties and operate alone; on the fringes of their mainstream peer group; or within a sub-group of similarly disassociated youth (9-12). In such instances, isolated adolescents typically endeavour to forge a new counter, non-conforming social identity. They do this through engaging in actions that bring them to the attention of both their mainstream and non-mainstream peers. A common means of forging a non-conforming deviant identity is to engage in progressively risky acts of anti-sociality (e.g., graffiti writing, binge drinking, drug taking, hoon driving, breaking and entry, robbery).

Success in these types of activities is determined, in part, by the amount of attention/respect such deviant actions garner from peers, as peer recognition not only affords the non-conforming perpetrator with an element of notoriety, but overtime also results in their attainment of a non-conforming social identity and inclusion in a non-conforming sub-group of likeminded peers (13). Therefore, it is through the formation of deviant friendships that aspiring youth are able to attain a non-conforming social identity and solidify their place within their selected non-conforming sub-group (14). However, the committing of deviant acts does not necessarily always result in the attainment of a non-conforming social identity or inclusion in a non-conforming sub-group. In such cases, adolescents who, either through choice or through circumstance, fail to gain peer recognition and/or sub-group acceptance tend to become social isolates (loners), socially disassociated from their mainstream and non-mainstream peers (7-8).

This outlined adolescent identity seeking process is consistent with Reputation Enhancement Theory, which over the years has become one of the foremost theories used to explain why adolescents engage in delinquent acts (4). The theory's main premise is that adolescent behaviour is largely motivated by a desire to present in a certain manner so as to gain peer recognition and social approval (15-16). In order to attain approval from mainstream peers adolescents behave in ways that are consistent with the personal identity they are trying to portray and with the prevailing collective identity and social mores of their mainstream peers. Moreover, peer evaluation of their performance not only dictates their full, partial, peripheral or non-acceptance within the mainstream peer-group, but also what social status is subsequently afforded them. Therefore, the need to obtain peer recognition is all important to adolescents, regardless of whether they are trying to establish a law-abiding conforming reputation or whether they are trying to establish a non-conforming deviant reputation. In the case of adolescents seeking a non-conforming deviant reputation there is the added pressure to provide both their mainstream and non-mainstream peers with public proof of their acts of daring (7, 17). Driven by this pressure, non-conforming adolescents are placed in the position of continually having to 'up-the-anti' if they are to maintain their non-conforming deviant identity.

Recent investigations into the motivations of adolescents for engaging in the most common entry level act of anti-social daring, graffiti tagging, indicates that mainstream peer recognition is largely achieved through the adolescent taggers' displayed ability to place tags in positions of visual prominence (13). While most graffiti tagging is done by adolescents sneaking around the streets at night more 'street' kudos is given to those adolescents whose tag placements involve a degree of danger (e.g., tagging a moving object, tagging in the open during daylight hours, or hanging upside down to tag a bridge span) (18). By engaging in such high-risk acts adolescent taggers also attract the attention of deviant like-minded peers. However, it is the 'street proof' of their ability to project a sustained visible presence on the streets that gains them the necessary recognition (props) from their peers to both attain the prized graffiti writer social identity as well as invites to join (dropped into) established graffiti crews (13, 19). It is through their association with established crew members that 'toy' (inexperienced) adolescent taggers are able to develop and refine their writing-style design skills. While considerable research effort has been directed towards understanding the negative scholastic implications of poor peer-group affirmation in early adolescence (9-10), insufficient research effort to date has been devoted to understanding the socialization patterns of deviant adolescents pursuing a non-conforming *graffiti-writer* social identity.

In Australia, the Western Australian 2005 state crime statistics and the Australian Institute of Criminology's 2004 federal justice statistics reveal graffiti tagging to be one of the most common acts of anti-social daring engaged in by adolescents aged 13-17 years. Moreover, that the general offending rate for adolescents is approximately five times higher than that of the whole Australian offending population (7). Though, in reality this figure may be a considerable underestimation of the prevalence of adolescent offending as the actions of many juvenile offenders are never recorded in juvenile justice statistics (20). Recent research has demonstrated that graffiti-writing is for prolific writers a gateway crime towards more serious offending (21).

While Reputation Enhancement Theory provides a social developmental framework for understanding the psychology behind the actions of adolescents seeking a non-conforming graffiti-writer social identity, much more research is needed to develop an in-depth understanding of the socialization practices of adolescent graffiti taggers (i.e., where and with whom they 'hang out'). Furthermore, it is interesting to note that the peak age range of graffiti offending (i.e., 13-15 years) coincides with the age range identified as being critical to adolescent identity formation (6, 22).

Other insights into the identity establishment practices of adolescent graffiti crew affiliates/members can be gleaned from studying the parallel body of literature pertaining to youth gang research. For instance, it is known that American and British youth gangs characteristically provide their gang members with social capital support resources. At an individual and at a collective level this support enables gang members to become efficient offenders (23-24). It has also been determined that while some youth gangs operate over an extensive geographic area other youth gangs operate in relatively localized areas (25). At present, comparatively little is known about the territoriality of individual graffiti-writers and graffiti crews, or the level of support they provide to their membership. In this regard, the presented exploratory study addresses this knowledge shortfall by exploring the territorial 'practices of prolific graffiti taggers through examining the placement location of their tags. This examination is conducted in two stages. First, in Stage 1, frequency tally counts are compiled to identify prolific taggers operating within the boundaries of an inner city locale within Perth, the state capital city of Western Australia. In Stage 2, the recorded tags of 16 prolific taggers are plotted on individual square street grid plots. These plots are then overlaid to reveal the prolific taggers' patterns of association.

OUR STUDY

Permission was sought and granted from the governing university's Human Ethics Committee for the presented study. Within the state of Western Australia the collection of documentary evidence of graffiti images is largely conducted through the auspices of public and privately funded graffiti removal contractors. This documentary evidence, however, is not uniformly collected. For example, some removalists in some council jurisdictions prior to removal take photographic evidence of all of the graffiti images they clean off and, complete a standardised Police Graffiti Report Form. The form details (among other things) the date and time of the image's removal, the location of the image, a description of the surface damage, the cost associated with the removal of the image, the colour of the image, the implement used by the offender, and a description of what has been written. Copies of the completed form and the photographic images are then sent electronically by the removalist to the contracting city council, who in turn, forwards the removalist's documentation to police for inclusion in their offender data base. However, other Western Australian city councils, discouraged by a perceived lack of progress in reducing the proliferation of graffiti, instruct their graffiti removal contractors to simply submit a bulk billing demand for their removal work, thus eliminating the need to engage in the more costly practice of compiling documentary evidence.

Given the inconsistency in documentation collection and time and costs limitations, the research team decided to randomly select one set of records from a pool of eight sets of removal records supplied to the researchers by eight city councils using the electronic image capture method of record keeping. The selected council's image and documentary records were then subjected to visual inspection, frequency distribution analysis and square grid plotting. These procedures are detailed in turn.

Frequency distribution analysis

A total of 1,462 police report forms were scrutinized and their attached images indexed. From this scrutiny a total of 2,729 discernible tags were identified. Of these 2,729 tags approximately half were multiple recordings of the same tag (e.g., 121 recordings of the *Blot* tag occurred on a variety of different structures over the study's three month record keeping period). Through this visual checking procedure it was possible to identify 1,072 different tag names, each of which was entered into an Excel spreadsheet. Through this recording procedure it was soon apparent that some of the 1,072 tag names had a root tag name plus multiple derivations. For example, the root tag name *Blot* appears in the following derivations, *Blots, Blotz, Blotzr, Blotsr,* and *Blotsa*. To determine the likely ownership of root tag names and their associated derivations, six known graffitists and six Police graffiti intelligence officers from across Australia were contacted and asked to give an opinion of the likely ownership of root and derivative tag names. Each interviewee was asked whether in their experience a tag derivation such as *Blotsa* was likely to be an extension of the *Blot* root tag and, as such, would belong to *Blot*. While none of the interviewees could definitively say that every appearance of a root tag (e.g., *Blot)* or one of its many derivations would have been personally written by the root tag owner (i.e., *Blot*) and not by a crew member 'putting it up' for *Blot,* the consensus of opinion was that in most instances root tag names such as *Blot* and their multiple derivations are likely to be 'owned' by one and the same graffiti tagger. The reason given for this summation was that taggers generally own one or more root tags and while they sometime use derivations of their root tag(s) and while other taggers sometimes put up their root tag(s) (or one of their derivations) for them, they do not consistently do so because it diminishes their own ability to either establish/maintain their own street identity. Given that the 'putting up' limitation could apply to each of the study's identified 1,072 tags it was decided to proceed with the examination based on the interview consensus that a root tag and its multiple associated derivations are characteristically owned by one individual. Working from this premise, the originally identified 1,072 tag names were reduced to 759 individual tag owners. A frequency tally was conducted of the number of occurrences of each of the 759 tags over the three month study period. Visual inspection of the final tally revealed that the majority of the tags belonged to 16 highly prolific taggers (11 of whom had a root tag name plus multiple derivations). These prolific taggers accounted for approximately 50% (n=1,373) of the total 2,729 recorded tags.

In order, to de-identify the street names of the 16 prolific taggers each of their root tag names have been ascribed a pseudo tag name. Finally, using the compiled Excel frequency tally, percentages were calculated to determine the number of times each tagger's tag had been photographically captured in isolation from tags belonging to each of the other 15 prolific taggers and, in addition, the number of times each tagger's tag had been photographically captured in close proximity to a tag belonging to one of the other 15 prolific taggers.

Square grid plots

To determine the extent of each of the 16 prolific taggers' tagging territory each documented tag location of each tagger's tag was plotted onto an individualized 11x14 street square grid plot which covered the area of the studied council's jurisdiction. To de-identify the participant council's data set all 14 streets running parallel to the X axis on the grid block were ascribed a number and a street suffix (i.e., 1-14th Street) depending on their relative position on the grid and similarly all 11 streets running parallel to the Y axis of the grid were numbered and ascribed an Avenue suffix (i.e., 1-11th Ave). Using this grid block system it was possible to position each recorded tag's location within one of the grids 154 squares. The use of square grid plots (graticules) is a standard geographic technique used for analysing high density location specific data with a non-random distribution (25).

FINDINGS

Stage 1: A tally of the 1,373 tags written by the study's prolific taggers is presented in Table 1. The table clearly reveals that even within this study's comparatively small cohort of 16 prolific taggers considerable activity variation exists. For example, five of the prolific taggers (i.e., *Blot, Done, Push, Ikan, & Zap*) each wrote in excess of a hundred tags; six prolific taggers (i.e., *Enter, Foxt, Krate, Legit, Must & Testr*) each wrote between 75-99 tags; and the remaining five prolific taggers (i.e., *Hate, Ole, Rsist, Send & Vile*) each wrote between 41-74 tags.

The bolded numbers in Table 1 indicate the number of times each individual tagger's tag was photographed in isolation (i.e., not in adjoining proximity to a tag written by one of the other 15 identified prolific taggers). The non-bolded numbers indicate the number of times each individual prolific tagger's tag was found in adjoining proximity to a tag belonging to one of the other 15 identified prolific taggers.

Percentages of the number of times each prolific tagger's tag was found in isolation from and in adjoining proximity to the tags of any of the other 15 prolific taggers were calculated and are presented in Table 2.

Visual inspection of Table 2 reveals that only one prolific tagger (i.e., *Ole*) spent more than half (i.e., 52%) of the time engaged in placing his/her tag in sites isolated from those frequented by the other 15 prolific taggers. Four of the other 15 prolific taggers (i.e., *Push* [27%], *Legit* [33%], *Rsist* [34%], & *Done* [38%]) each spent approximately a third of their tagging time placing tags in isolated locations. While ten prolific taggers (i.e., *Blot* [79%], *Enter* [75%], *Foxt* [84%], *Hate* [77%], *Krate [*86%], *Must* [80%], *Send* [83%], *Testr* [87.5%], *Ikan* [83%] & *Zap* [77%]) spent between 75-87.5% of their tagging time placing tags in adjoining proximity to one or more of the tags belonging to the other 15 prolific taggers. Only one tagger (i.e., *Vile*, [94%]) spent almost all of his/her tagging time writing tags on sites frequented by the other 15 prolific taggers. By further calculating the percentage of times each of the study's 16 prolific taggers' tags were captured in close proximity to each other it was possible to establish which taggers frequently tagged together (see Table 3).

Table 1. Frequency count of times each individual tagger's tags appeared in isolation (figure in bold) and in close proximity to each one of the other 15 prolific taggers (non-bold figures)

	Blot	Done	Enter	Foxt	Hate	Krate	Legit	Must	Ole	Push	Rsist	Send	Testr	Vile	Ikan	Zap	Total
Blot	**25**	6	9	8	4	8	7	9	1	10	1	4	6	4	9	10	121
Done		**39**	5	5	5	3	4	4	4	6	1	1	5	5	5	5	103
Enter			**24**	5	2	5	5	5	1	9	2	3	6	1	6	7	95
Foxt				**16**	4	6	6	7	2	8	1	3	7	3	7	9	97
Hate					**15**	2	4	3	4	3	3	0	3	5	4	4	65
Krate						**11**	5	5	1	7	1	3	5	2	7	8	79
Legit							**32**	3	0	6	2	2	5	2	7	7	97
Must								**16**	0	4	2	2	5	3	6	5	79
Ole									**31**	1	5	0	3	2	3	2	60
Push										**34**	1	5	7	3	10	10	124
Rsist											**15**	0	3	2	3	2	44
Send												**7**	3	1	3	4	41
Testr													**11**	3	7	9	88
Vile														**3**	4	4	47
Ikan															**18**	10	109
Zap																**28**	124
																	1,373

Table 2. Percentage of times each individual prolific tagger's total tag frequency count that appeared in isolation (by self) or in close proximity to a tag belonging to one or more of the other 15 prolific taggers

Prolific taggers	% of tagging conducted alone	% of tagging conducted in the presence of others
Blot	21	79
Done	38	62
Enter	25	75
Foxt	16	84
Hate	23	77
Krate	14	86
Legit	33	67
Must	20	80
Ole	**52**	**48**
Push	27	73
Rsist	34	66
Send	17	83
Testr	12.5	87.5
Vile	6	94
Ikan	17	83
Zaps	23	77

Each taggers tagging preference for tagging alone or tagging with one or more of the other prolific taggers is clearly discernable from Table 3. For instance, *Ole, Done, Hate, & Rsist* tag in adjoining proximity to each other 13-17% of the time while *Send's* tag is rarely (i.e., less than 5% of the time) found near the tags of *Hate, Ole, Rsist* or *Vile.*

*Stage 2:*In order, to identify the extent of the overlap between the tagging territories of taggers who often write their tags in positions of adjoining proximity, the location of each of the 16 taggers' captured tags were plotted onto an individual 11 x 14 street square grid plot according to the removalists' documented image location address. By photocopying each grid plot onto a transparency and overlaying the transparencies it was possible to identify the location of territorial tagging hubs (see Table 4 for a simplified example of the overlay transparency street square grid plots for taggers *Ole, Done, Hate, Rsist, Testr & Ikan*).

Finally, visual inspection of all 16 prolific taggers' tagging territory grid plots revealed the existence of three distinct tagging activity patterns (see Table 5).

First, a *compact* pattern exists where taggers confine the placement of their tags to a relatively limited number of streets. Second, an *interlinking* pattern of tagging exists where tags are placed in adjoining streets. Third, a *scattered* tagging pattern exists where taggers place their tags in a disperse area of disconnected streets.

Table 3. Percentage of times that each prolific tagger's tag was electronically captured in close proximity to each of the other prolific taggers' tags

	Blot	Done	Enter	Foxt	Hate	Krate	Legit	Must	Ole	Push	Rsist	Send	Testr	Vile	Ikan	Zap
	%	%	%	%	%	%	%	%	%	%	%	%	%	%	%	%
Blot	x	6	9	8	4	8	7	9	1	10	1	4	6	4	9	10
Done	6	x	8	8	8	5	6	6	6	9	2	2	8	8	8	8
Enter	12	7	x	7	3	7	7	7	1	12	3	4	8	1	8	10
Foxt	10	6	6	x	5	7	7	9	2	10	1	4	9	4	9	11
Hate	8	10	4	8	x	4	8	6	8	6	6	0	6	10	8	8
Krate	12	4	7	9	3	x	7	7	1	10	1	4	7	3	10	12
Legit	11	6	8	9	6	8	x	4	0	9	3	3	8	3	11	11
Must	14	6	8	11	5	8	5	x	0	6	3	3	8	5	10	8
Ole	3	14	3	7	14	3	0	0	x	3	17	0	10	7	10	7
Push	11	7	10	9	3	8	7	4	1	x	1	6	8	3	11	11
Rsist	3	3	7	3	10	3	7	7	17	3	x	0	10	7	10	7
Send	12	3	9	9	0	9	6	6	0	15	0	x	9	3	9	12
Testr	8	6	8	9	4	6	6	6	4	9	4	4	x	4	9	12
Vile	9	11	2	7	11	5	5	7	5	7	5	2	7	x	9	9
Ikan	10	5	7	8	4	8	8	7	3	11	3	3	8	4	x	11
Zap	10	5	7	9	4	8	7	5	2	10	2	4	9	4	10	x

17-13% of time	Frequently tag together
12-9% of time	Often tag together
8-5% of time	Infrequently tag together
4-0 % of time	Rarely if ever tag together

Table 4. Overlay of five prolific taggers (*Ole, Done, Hate, Rsist, Testr* & *Ikan*) territorial grid box plots

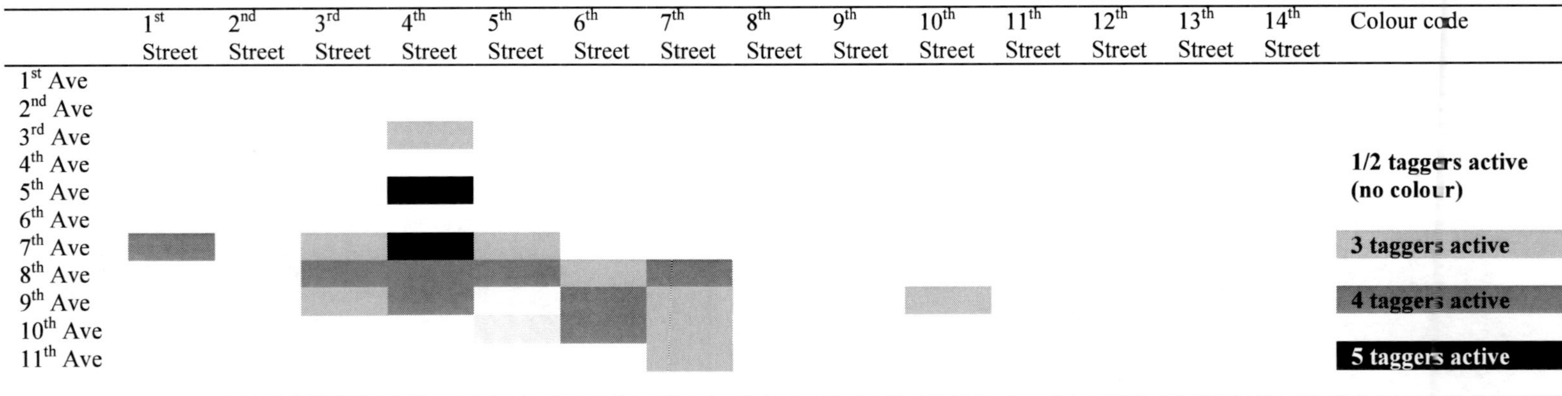

Table 5. Territorial tagging activity patterns of prolific graffiti offenders

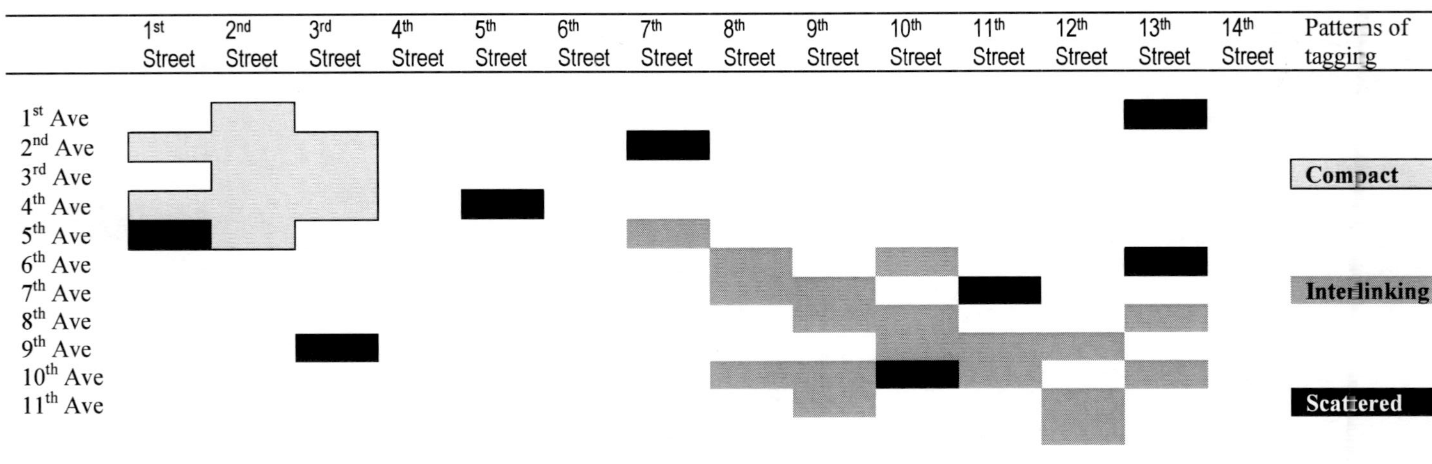

Discussion

This research begins to fill a current void in the understanding of the socialization and territorial tagging practices of prolific graffiti taggers. In this regard, the research has exposed three aspects of their socialization practices. First, the research has shown that considerable variation exists in the number of times prolific taggers engage in the act of graffiti tagging. For example five prolific taggers wrote in excess of 100 tags over a three month recording period, six prolific taggers wrote between 75-99 tags and five prolific taggers wrote between 41-75 tags. So this raises the question: Why are some prolific taggers more prolific than other prolific taggers? Given that all of the 1,373 prolifically written tags were all written on similar street level stationary structures it is unlikely that any of these prolifically written tags accrued a dissimilar amount of street kudos. Therefore, it is posited that the tag frequency variations evidenced in this study are linked (amongst other factors) to the taggers' recognised level of tag writing proficiency and motivational desire/need to maintain a visible street presence. For instance, it may well be that prolific taggers writing the highest number of tags are individuals trying to establish a street identity through the process of 'bombing' an area with tags and, thus, attaining maximum tag visual recognition amongst their peers. Or conversely, it could also be posited that the most prolific taggers were experienced taggers actively marking out an area of tagging turf. While either of these posited scenarios sit within Hitchcock's (1) adolescence 'identity crisis' theory and the thesis of Reputation Enhancement (4) they do not enhance understanding of the identity-seeking motivations of the least active members of the identified cohort of prolific taggers. In this latter case, it is plausible to hypothesise that prolific taggers writing the least number of tags are either 'apprenticed' taggers learning the 'graffiti trade' or are established taggers writing the smallest number of tags necessary to maintain a street presence. Clearly, these opposing possible interpretations highlight the need for further research into the motivational forces behind the writing practices of prolific graffiti taggers.

The second aspect of the prolific taggers' tagging practices to emerge from the present study is that tagging at the prolific level is predominantly a group activity, in so far as 15 individuals from the cohort of 16 prolific taggers spent the majority of their tagging time writing tags in close proximity to one or more of the other identified prolific taggers. This finding is consistent with Reputation Enhancement Theory which contends that the adolescent identity establishment process requires young people to provide to their peers visible proof of their daring (17).

Elmer and Reicher (16) also hypothesize that the act of bestowal of a non-conforming social identity by like-minded deviant peers to a new entrant to the group/sub-culture actually provides both the newcomer and the bestowing group of delinquent peers with a certain degree of mutually beneficial protective social capital. Warr (26) posits that the adolescent need for such protective social capital resources actually increases when non-conforming adolescents widen their social interactional base. Indeed, it is reasoned that their wider interaction with deviant peers significantly increases the likelihood of physical confrontation.

Thus, increased social visibility, shared behavioural inclinations and physical rivalries are the necessary grist for the adolescent reputation enhancement non-conforming social identity mill. Hence, deviant adolescents seeking a non-conforming social identity are posited to be motivated by a non-conforming adolescent desire for peer recognition and peer-group status.

However, much more research is needed to refine the present understanding of why some taggers choose to tag in close proximity and in full view of their peers while others prefer to tag predominantly on their own. Cordin (27) and Houghton et al. (7) argue that one reason for this seeming dichotomy might well be that adolescents who engage in private acts of deviance might harbour a reputational desire to be viewed as neither conforming or non-conforming in public, yet privately, harbour a desire to be non-conforming.

Research into the persistence and desistence offending trajectories of adolescents suggests, however, that some degree of public and private offending during adolescence is commonplace, normative and in many instances relatively temporary (7, 28-29). Moreover, the body of youth persistence and desistence literature delineates four offending trajectories (see 6, 29-32). Namely, the early-onset childhood life course persister who continues to offend well into adulthood; the early-onset childhood limited desister who ceases offending before obtaining adulthood; the late-onset adolescent persister who continues to offend into adulthood; and the late-onset adolescent limited desister who ceases offending before obtaining adulthood. With regard to taggers who tag in the company of others versus taggers who tag on their own it has yet to be determined whether these two types of taggers are most commonly situated in one or more of these four youth offending trajectories.

The third and final insight into the practices of prolific graffiti taggers to emerge from the present study pertains to the finding that taggers 'hang-out' in hubs. In addition, that the taggers who hang-out in hubs display three distinct patterns of tagging, namely, a *compact*, an *interlinking*, and a *scattered* pattern. The study's hypothesise that taggers hangout in hubs partly in order to socialize and partly to engage in shared tagging activities is consistent with both Reputation Enhancement Theory and the body of adolescent deviance literature which both suggest that a clear correlation exists between the adolescent inclination to engage in delinquent activities in order to gain a desired reputation and their friends' inclination to engage in delinquent activities to maintain a non-conforming reputation (4, 33).

In conclusion, the present study, based on the thesis Reputation Enhancement Theory, has provided some initial insights into the socialization activities of adolescent graffiti taggers. Though, further research is now needed to solidify and extend the current findings so that advances can be made both in the construction of effective social intervention programs for non-conforming youth engaged in graffiti tagging. Particularly so if meaningful progress is to be made in re-integrating offenders back into mainstream society through converting their non-conforming reputational desires back into conforming reputational desires.

REFERENCES

[1] Hitchcock J. Adolescent gang participation: Psychological perspectives. J Police Crim Psych 2001;16:33-47.

[2] Taylor MF, Houghton S, Bednall J. Friendships, peer socialization and social identity among adolescent skateboarders and graffiti writers. New York: Nova Science, 2010.

[3] Erikson EH. Childhood and society. NY: WW Norton,1993.

[4] Carroll AM, Houghton S, Durkin K, Hattie J. Adolescent reputations and risk: developmental trajectories to delinquency. Bloomington: Springer, 2009.

[5] Durkin K, Houghton S. Children's and adolescents' stereotypes of tattooed people as delinquent. Leg Crim Psych 2000;5:153-64.

[6] Carroll AM, Hemingway F, Bower J, Ashman A, Houghton S, Durkin K. Impulsivity in juvenile delinquency: Differences among early-onset, late-onset, and non-offenders. J Youth Adolesc 2006;35:519-29.
[7] Houghton S, Carroll A, Tan C, Hopkins S. Self-reported delinquency and reputational orientations of high school and incarcerated adolescent loners and non-loners. J Forensic Psych Psych2008;19:205-27.
[8] Taylor MF, Houghton S. Initiating and sustaining peer friendships: socialization patterns of students diagnosed with an attentional disorder. Br J Spec Ed 2008;35:209-19.
[9] Buhs ES, Ladd GW. Peer rejection in kindergarten as an antecedent of young children's social adjustment: An examination of mediating processes. Dev Psychol 2001;37:550-60.
[10] Buhs ES, Ladd GW, Herald SL. Peer exclusion and victimization: processes that meditate the relation between peer group rejection and children's classroom engagement and achievement? J Educ Psychol 2006;98:1-13.
[11] Ladd GW, Kochenderfer BJ, Coleman CC. Classroom peer acceptance, friendship, and victimization: distant relational systems that contribute uniquely to children's school adjustment? Child Dev 1997;68:1181-97.
[12] Sunwolf LL. Being left out: rejecting outsiders and communicating group boundaries in childhood and adolescent peer groups. J Appl Commun Res 2004;32:195-23.
[13] Taylor MF. Addicted to the risk, recognition and respect that the graffiti lifestyle provides: Towards an understanding of the reasons for graffiti engagement. Int J Ment Health Addict 2012;10:54-68.
[14] Goodnight JA, Bates JE, Newman JP, Dodge KA, Pettit GS. The interactive influences of friend deviance and reward dominance on the development of externalizing behaviour during middle adolescence. J Abnorm Child Psych 2006;34:573-583.
[15] Agnew R. The interactive effects of peer variables on delinquency. Criminology1991;2:47-72.
[16] Emler N, Reicher SD. Adolescence and delinquency: The collective management of
[17] reputation. Cambridge, MA: Blackwell, 1995.
[18] Elmer N. Differential involvement in delinquency: Towards an interpretation in terms of
[19] reputation management. In: Mahler BA, Maher WB. Progress in experimental personality research. New York: Acad Press, 1984.
[20] Taylor MF, Houghton S. The Singaporean solution in the Western Australian context: Reputation enhancement – A model for understanding graffiti proliferation. Paper presented at the meeting of the Institute of Public Works Engineering Australia, Fremantle, Australia, 2008.
[21] Taylor MF, Marais I. Does urban art deter graffiti proliferation? An evaluation of an Australian commissioned urban art project. Papers British Criminol Conf 2009;9:57-70.
[22] Maxfield MG, Weiler BL, Widom CS. Comparing self-reports and official records of arrests. J Quant Crim 2000;16:87-110.
[23] Taylor MF, Marais I, Cottman R. Patterns of graffiti offending: towards recognition that graffiti offending is more than 'kids messing around'. Policing Soc 2012;22:152-168.
[24] Loh NS, Maller MG, Fernandez JA, Ferrante AM, Walsh MR. 2007 Crime and justice statistics for Western Australia. URL: htpp://www.crc.law.uwa.edu.au
[25] Deuchar R. Gangs, marginalised youth and social capital. Stoke-on-Trent, UK: Trentham Books, 2009.
[26] Tita G, Ridgeway G. The impact of gang formation on local patterns of crime. J Res Crime Delinquency 2007;44:208-37.
[27] Block R. Gang activity and overall levels of crime: A new mapping tool for defining areas of gang activity using police records. J Quant Crim 2000;16:369-83.
[28] Warr M. Companions in crime: The social aspects of criminal conduct. Cambridge: Cambridge Univ Press, 2002.
[29] Cordin RM. Psychopathic-like traits in children and adolescents: Differential patterns and relationships with proactive and reactive aggression, and anxiety. Unpublished doc dissertation, Uni Western Australia, Perth, Australia, 2007.
[30] Moffitt TE. "Life-course-persistent" and "adolescence-limited" antisocial behaviour: A developmental taxonomy. Psychol Rev1993:100:674–701.

[31] Moffitt TE. Males on the life-course persistent and adolescence-limited antisocial pathways: Follow-up at age 26. Dev Psychopathol 2003;14:179-207.
[32] Burt SA, Mikolajewski AJ. Preliminary evidence that specific candidate genes are associated with adolescent-onset antisocial behaviour. Aggress Behav 2008;34:437-45.
[33] Chung IJ, Hill KG, Hawkins JD, Gilchrist LD, Nagin DS. Childhood predictors of offense trajectories. J Res Crime Delinquency 2002;39:60-90.
[34] Piquero AR, Chung HL. On the relationships between gender, early onset, and the seriousness of offending. J Criminal Justice 2001;29:189–206.
[35] Kreager DA. Strangers in the halls: Isolation and delinquency in school networks. Soc Forces 2004;83:351-90.

In: School, Adolescence and Health Issues
Editors: J. Merrick, A. Tenenbaum and H. A. Omar
ISBN: 978-1-62948-702-1

Chapter 10

KIDNEY TRANSPLANTS IN ADOLESCENCE

***Cheryl Belair, CCLS*[1], *Jordan Gilleland, PhD*[2,*] *and Sandra Amaral, MD, MHS*[3]**

[1]Department of Transplant Services, Children's Healthcare of Atlanta, Atlanta, Georgia, US

[2] Department of Pediatrics, Emory University School of Medicine, Atlanta, Georgia, US

[3]Department of Pediatrics, Perelman School of Medicine, University of Pennsylvania, Philadelphia, Pennsylvania, US

ABSTRACT

Adolescents with kidney transplants are at increased risk for allograft rejection and loss. These negative health outcomes are likely multifactorial, but seem to be exacerbated during the time of transition from pediatric to adult healthcare providers. In June 2007, our center initiated an adolescent-focused transition clinic for adolescent kidney transplant recipients with the goal of improving adolescent healthcare self-management and easing adolescents' transition to adult health services. We conducted a telephone survey of 21 young adult kidney transplant recipients who had attended this transition clinic to assess their satisfaction with receiving adolescent-specific, multidisciplinary care. Eleven patients (52%) had transitioned within the prior 2 years and 10 patients (48%) were pending transition in the coming year. All 21 patients felt that being seen independently was beneficial. Nineteen patients (90%) believed that the adolescent clinic helped them prepare for transition to the adult center and 18 patients (86%) felt more knowledgeable about their medical condition and disease after attending the clinic. Those that did not feel that the clinic helped them stated that they already felt knowledgeable about their medications and condition prior to the clinic. Nine of the eleven patients (82%) who had transferred noted that they felt fully prepared at time of transition. These results suggest that adolescents with kidney transplants perceive benefit from attending an adolescent-focused transition clinic. Whether improved health knowledge and

[*] Correspondence: Jordan Gilleland, PhD, Assistant Professor, Emory University School of Medicine, Department of Pediatrics, Children's Healthcare of Atlanta, 1405 Clifton Rd. NE, Aflac Cancer Center, 4th floor, Atlanta, GA, 30322-1060 United States. E-mail: Jordan.Gilleland@choa.org.

improved ability to communicate with providers independently leads to better long-term health outcomes and smoother transition deserves further exploration.

INTRODUCTION

Children who undergo kidney transplantation at less than 18 years of age experience excellent one-year allograft survival rates of 93-94%, however these statistics alarmingly change at 5 years status post transplant. The 5-year allograft survival rate for patients who receive a transplanted kidney between the ages of 11 and 17 years drops to a disappointing 63% (1). The only other age group to experience such a low allograft survival rate (59%) is comprised of patients over 65 years of age. In the North American Pediatric Renal Trials and Collaborative Studies (NAPRTCS) registry, adolescents had the poorest graft survival among all pediatric age groups, and once diagnosed with rejection, they did not respond as well to treatment, exhibiting fewer complete rejection reversals and greater residual allograft dysfunction (2).

These negative health outcomes in adolescents are likely multifactorial, but seem to be exacerbated during the time of transition from pediatric to adult healthcare providers (3-4). The transition of adolescents to adult medical services adds to the risk of allograft loss because of discontinuity in care combined with the complex and challenging psychosocial issues faced by adolescents with chronic illness. In a study of 20 young adults with kidney transplants in the United Kingdom who had been transferred from pediatric to adult transplant centers, 8 transplants failed within 36 months of transfer (40%) (4). In 2007, the United States Government Accountability Office published a report that examined the frequency of transplant failures and subsequent cost to Medicare from 1997 through 2004 (5). Three age groups were defined: pediatric recipients were those younger than 18 years old, transitional recipients were those younger than 18 at the time of transplant and at least 18 at the end of the study interval, and adult recipients were those at least 18 at the time of transplant. Transitional recipients experienced the highest rate of transplant failures compared with pediatric or adult recipients illustrating the challenges present during the adolescent years.

Medication nonadherence is a major risk factor for allograft rejection and loss in both adults and pediatrics and results in poor long-term kidney transplant outcomes and subsequent devastating medical and economic consequences on individual and societal levels. Ettenger et al. (6) found that nonadherence led to rejection with subsequent kidney allograft loss or dysfunction in 71% of patients who had received deceased donor kidney transplants (N=70). The UNOS registry has reported that 13% of allograft loss in adolescent kidney transplant recipients is due to nonadherence.[7] In a recent study of the USRDS database, Chisholm et al. (8) found that pediatric kidney transplant recipients who experienced allograft failure were twice as likely to be nonadherent (OR 2.07, 95% CI 1.12-4.06) and greater adherence to immunosuppressive medication was significantly associated with longer time to graft failure (P=0.009).

Although transition programming for adolescents with chronic illness is purported to be necessary, there is little evidence to support their utility. Two years after designing and implementing an Adolescent Kidney Transplant Transition Clinic (AKTTC), we performed survey of patients who attended our transition clinic and transitioned to or are pending transition to an adult healthcare setting within the year to assess patient satisfaction with such a comprehensive program. In the current investigation, we review participants' surveys to explore patient satisfaction with the AKTTC.

ADOLESCENT KIDNEY TRANSPLANT TRANSITION CLINIC

In June 2007, we initiated a novel Adolescent Kidney Transplant Transition Clinic (AKTTC) as a healthcare self-management program at Emory-Children's Healthcare of Atlanta. Healthcare self-management and the provision of transitional care are inextricably linked with medication adherence and are necessary components of caring for adolescents with chronic illness. At least one study in adolescent liver transplant recipients has demonstrated that an intervention designed to facilitate transition of healthcare responsibility from parent to patient can result in improved medication adherence (9). The Society for Adolescent Medicine, maintaining the belief that adolescents can be empowered to effect positive health-related outcomes, proposed transition principles for optimal health care services to facilitate the transition of adolescents with chronic illness to adult health care providers. These principles include providing age-appropriate care, enhancing autonomy, addressing adolescent-specific health issues, and designating particular health professionals to facilitate this process of development (10). In the development of the AKTTC at Emory-CHOA, we have modeled a unique healthcare self-management program that implements the principles of adolescent transition. Patients join the program when they turn 14 years old or reach one year post-transplant, when laboratory monitoring and visit frequency become less frequent and allograft survival rates begin to decline (11). The intensive multidisciplinary care team sees patients every three months. Patients rotate through 15-minute encounters with six different care providers, including the transplant coordinator, psychologist, social worker, pharmacist, nutritionist or child life specialist and a designated nephrologist. The nutritionist and child life specialist alternate seeing patients every other visit. Importantly, to reinforce the concept of the adolescent's autonomy and responsibility for self-care, patients are seen alone, while parents wait in the waiting room. Parents are then consulted at the end of the visit. Patients receive more one-on-one time for communication and counseling with each healthcare provider. Care providers incorporate several approaches to address adherence, including behavioral modification strategies and patient education. In our program, each provider asks the patient a pre-specified set of questions to identify facilitators and barriers to adherence. The patient interviews encourage frank discussion about the impact of individual behavior and environmental influences on overall health status and specifically allograft function. The clinical programming focuses on encouraging a development progression of responsibility of healthcare by the patient.

Each member of the care team has a specific role designed to achieve a 21-item checklist of healthcare self-management skills that we recommend patients achieve prior to transition to adult medical care, including such tasks as calling in one's own medication refills and carrying a medication list in one's wallet. This checklist is given to patients at their first clinic visit; the patient is assigned up to three tasks from this checklist as homework at the end of each visit and his/her progress toward achievement of these tasks is assessed at the next visit. The pharmacist is responsible for assessing the patient's medication knowledge, including medication indications and doses, as well as medication adherence and barriers to adherence.

The pharmacist and patient develop a plan for improvement in knowledge and adherence between visits. The transplant coordinator and physician deal with any medical issues as well as assess the patient's knowledge of his/her diagnosis, address sexual health, substance and alcohol use, and the impact of behavior on transplant function. The psychologist identifies and addresses any psychosocial co-morbidities which may impact adherence, such as depression or family conflict. The process of transition to adult services is discussed with the patient at each visit. Positive reinforcement is provided for improvements in healthcare self-management skills. To make further gains in healthcare self-management, behavioral strategies, such as programming medication reminder alarms into one's cell phone, are individually developed with each patient.

PATIENT SURVEY

For this survey, we telephoned any patient who was seen at least twice in the AKTTC program and who had transitioned to the adult healthcare setting or who was pending transition to the adult healthcare setting within the upcoming year. Patients were telephoned from January 11, 2010-February 11, 2010.

We based our clinic model on the principles of transition recommended by Rosen et al. (10), such as providing opportunities to enhance autonomy, increase personal responsibility and facilitate self reliance. Our survey questions were directed toward learning more about which components of our model were of most and least benefit from the patient perspective. The purpose was to assess our current efficacy in improving the transition of care from the patient's viewpoint and using the data to improve our multidisciplinary cared model beyond its current form. A preliminary review of this study was conducted by the Children's Healthcare of Atlanta/Emory University School of Medicine IRB Board and was deemed exempt from a full review due to its quality improvement nature.

The AKTTC satisfaction survey asked a series of twelve questions. Participant responses to questions 1-6 are detailed in table 2. To assess patients' opinions on clinic design and programming we asked: "Was meeting with the multidisciplinary team members independently, without parents, beneficial?", "Was seeing each team member at each clinic visit beneficial?", and "Where the homework assignments that you received in clinic beneficial?" To gauge perceptions of potential clinic benefits we asked: "Do you feel that the AKTTC helped prepare you for transition to the adult center?" and "Did you feel more knowledgeable about your medical condition and medication after attending the AKTTC?" and "Where there any differences between the pediatric transplant clinic and the adult clinic that you did not feel prepared for?"

The results of Questions 7-12 are not listed in table 2, but are listed in the body of this study. These questions asked patients to explain what part of the AKTTC helped them the most and least, changes to the AKTTC that they would recommend, how their kidney function is doing now, and what they are doing with their time. Clinical and medical characteristics, including age, race, gender and kidney transplant status were collected from the medical chart and are detailed in table 1. Survey responses were recorded verbatim.

FINDINGS

Twenty-five patients were eligible to participate in the survey. We were able to contact 22 patients by phone and 21 completed the telephone survey (95%). One patient declined participation. Of the patients who completed the survey, 33% were Black, 67% White, 67% male. Mean age was 21.1 years (± .75 years). Patients were seen on average 6.57 times (± 2.84 visits) in the AKTTC prior to transfer. Eleven patients (52%) had transferred to adult services. Ten (48%) will be transferring to adult services within the next year. Independent samples t-test were used to compare the pre- and post- transition participants. The pre-transition participants were significantly younger than the post-transition participants (t=-3.95, p=.002) and had attended significantly more AKTTC visits (t=4.69, p=.001).

Table 1. Demographics by group

Demographics	Pre-Transition Patients (N=10)	Post-Transition Patients (N=11)
Mean Age (years)* Age difference: t=-3.95 (p=.002)	20.60 (± .302)	21.57 (± .744)
Gender (N) Male Female	 8 (80.0%) 2 (20.0%)	 6 (54.4%) 5 (45.5%)
Ethnicity (N) Caucasian African American	 8 (80.0%) 2 (20.0%)	 6 (54.4%) 5 (45.5%)
Diagnosis (N) Cystic/Hereditary/Congenital Glomerulonephritis Secondary GN/Vasculitis Interstitial Nephritis/Pyelonephritis Miscellaneous	 1 (10%) 5 (50%) 2 (20%) 2 (20%) 0 (0%)	 2 (18.2%) 4 (36.4%) 2 (18.2%) 1 (9.1%) 2 (18.2%)
Mean Time since transplant (years)	6.30 (± 3.50)	5.65 (± 2.63)
Mean Age at transplant (years)	14.22 (± 3.38)	15.94 (± 2.69)
Mean Number of AKTTC visits* Visit number difference: t=4.69 (p=.001)	8.70 (± .1.41)	4.64 (± .2.38)

Among the 21 subjects who completed the survey, eighteen (86%) still had a functioning kidney transplant at the time they were surveyed. Two patients lost their transplant due to nonadherence but both cases occurred prior to transition to adult services. One additional patient lost allograft function after transition, however allograft loss occurred secondary to other medical complications, not related to adherence.

Table 2 provides a summary of survey responses. There were no significant differences in the survey answers of the pre- and post-transition groups. All 21patients found attending the AKTTC without his/her parents to be beneficial. The most common reasons for this were that the adolescents felt like they could share more information when the parents were not in the room and that they felt like they had more responsibility for their healthcare management. A few teens stated that they felt they had to change their answers to questions when their parents were present.

Table 2. Comparison of post transition patient and pre-transition patient responses to the AKTTC satisfaction survey

Question		Responses			Total
		Yes	No	Somewhat	
1. "Was meeting with the multidisciplinary team members independently, without parents, beneficial to you?"	Post-transition group Pre-transition group	8 7	- -	3 3	11 10
2. "Was seeing all of the team members at each clinic visit beneficial to you?"	Post-transition group Pre-transition group	10 8	1 2	- -	11 10
3. "Where the homework assignments that you received at each clinic visit beneficial to you?" **	Post-transition group Pre-transition group	4 5	- -	2 5	6 10
4. "Do you feel that the clinic helped prepare you for transitioning to the adult transplant center?"	Post-transition group Pre-transition group	7 6	1 1	3 3	11 10
5. "Did you feel more knowledgeable about your medical condition and medications after attending the ATTC clinic?"	Post-transition group Pre-transition group	5 9	2 1	4 -	11 10
6. "Where there any differences between the pediatric transplant clinic and the adult clinic that you did not feel prepared for?"	Post-transition group Pre-transition group	2 NA	9 NA	- NA	11 NA

Note: ** Five participants did not remember the homework assignments.

As part of the clinic programming, patients received homework assignments as detailed in the methods section. Sixteen patients (76%) remembered their homework assignments. Of those patients, the assignments that were believed to be most beneficial were learning medications and learning details about insurance.

Five patients (45%) toured the adult healthcare facility to which they would be transferring prior to their transfer. All 5 patients found this to be helpful because they knew where to go for clinic appointments and where able to meet the new staff. Four patients also remembered receiving a transition packet and contact info for the adult setting. Patients reported this to be beneficial and an easy place to find contact information when needed.

Eighteen patients (86%) felt that the AKTTC helped them prepare for transition to the adult center, by "learning to become independent in a step by step process". The three subjects who did not feel the AKTTC helped them be more prepared reported feeling well-prepared for transition prior to enrollment in the AKTTC. Eighteen patients (86%) reported that they felt more knowledgeable about their medical condition and their medications because of participation in the AKTTC program. Patients reported that the most helpful component of the program was meeting with all of the providers one on one, homework assignments, seeing the doctor independently and going on the tour. Of the eleven patients who had transferred to the adult setting, the biggest differences between the pediatric and adult settings were reported to be longer clinic visits and wait times, more responsibilities, and having to initiate concerns. Nine patients (81%) stated that they felt prepared to transition to the adult center at time of transfer. Of the 2 that did not feel prepared, they felt unprepared for "people's lack of helpfulness" at the adult center and "nurses are not as hands on" at the adult center.

CONCLUSION

Long-term allograft survival in adolescents with kidney transplants is poor and likely due to a myriad of reasons, including the complex developmental issues of adolescence with changes in independence, exacerbated by the transition of healthcare responsibility and transition of medical care from pediatric to adult healthcare settings. Transitional care is purported to be necessary to improve long-term health outcomes for adolescents with chronic illness but little is known regarding whether such programs are actually perceived to be beneficial by the patient. We initiated a multidisciplinary, adolescent-focused transitional care program based on the recommended principles of transition suggested by the Society for Adolescent Medicine. Patients who participated in this programming were surveyed and overall reported satisfaction with the AKTTC program. They also found it useful to meet the adult healthcare team in advance of their transfer. Further, both groups of patients pre-and post- transition reported experiencing equal benefits from the AKTTC programming which indicate that the advantages offered by the program are evident during the process of transition and after transfer of care. Our findings suggest that this type of program is worthwhile. Specifically, patients perceived benefit in meeting with providers independently, receiving adolescent specific education and being given more responsibility for management of their healthcare.

Our findings are consistent with those reported in other adolescent chronic illness populations. Several studies have reported the importance of patients being seen independently in the pediatric healthcare setting prior to transfer. Being seen independently has been associated with successful transfer in young adults with congenital heart disease, juvenile idiopathic arthritis, cystic fibrosis and other solid organ transplants (12-15). Patients with chronic illness have reported that the keys to successful transition include having transition be a stepwise process, having a trusting, reciprocal relationship with the healthcare team, including discussions about insurance and bridging differences between adult and pediatric healthcare settings (16). In addition, patients with varied chronic illnesses have reported that it is helpful to discuss transition early and to meet the adult healthcare team before transfer (17, 18). Taken together, the data suggest that it is likely a dynamic balance between adolescent healthcare responsibility and parental involvement during the transition process in which teens take on increasing amounts of responsibility and parents become less involved over time as teen's approach transfer to adult care.

Of the eleven patients that transitioned to the adult transplant clinic, only one patient (9%) returned to dialysis after transition and this was not related to nonadherence or loss to follow-up during transition. Of the patients who are impending transition to adult services from the pediatric setting, all feel more prepared for the transition as a result of receiving adolescent-focused and healthcare self-management focused care. Further study is warranted to assess long-term health outcomes of patients who attend an adolescent-focused transition clinic compared with those who do not receive such services.

ACKNOWLEDGEMENTS

The adolescent kidney transplant transition clinic at Emory-CHOA has been supported by The Mason Trust, The Georgia Transplant Foundation, Emory Healthcare and Children's Healthcare of Atlanta.

REFERENCES

[1] US Dept of HHS. UNOS: Organ Donation and Transplantation. 2010. URL: http://www.unos.org/data.

[2] Smith J, et al. Renal transplant outcomes in adolescents: A report of the North American Pediatric Renal Transplant Cooperative Study. Pediatr Transplant 2002;6(6):493-9.

[3] Annunziato R, et al. Adherence and medical outcomes in pediatric liver transplant recipients who transition to adult services. Pediatr Transplantation 2007;11(6):608-14.

[4] Watson A. Non-compliance and transfer from paediatric to adult transplant unit. Ped Nephrol 2000;14(6): 469-72.

[5] General Accountability Office. End-stage renal disease: Characteristics of kidney transplant recipients, Frequency of transplant failures, and cost to medicare. September 2007. GAO-07-1117.

[6] Ettenger R, et al. Improved cadaveric renal transplant outcomes in children. Pediatr Nephrol 1991;5(1):137-42.

[7] Cecka J, et al. Pediatric renal transplantation: a review of the UNOS data. Pediatr Transplant 1997;1(1):55-64.

[8] Chisholm-Burns MA, Spivey CA, et al. Immunosuppressant Therapy Adherence and Graft Failure Among Pediatric Renal Transplant Recipients. Am J Transplant 2009;9(11):2497-504.

[9] Annunziato R, et al. Transitioning health care responsibility from caregiver to patient: a pilot study aiming to facilitate medication adherence during this process. Ped Transpl 2008;12(3):309-15.

[10] Rosen D, et al. Transition to adult health care for adolescents and young adults with chronic conditions: Position paper of the Society for Adolescent Medicine. J Adolesc Health 2003;33(4):309-11.

[11] US Dept of Health and Human Services. United States OPTN/SRTR 2006 Annual Report. URL: http://www.optn.org/

[12] Reid GJ, Irvine MJ, McCrindle BW, Sananes R, Ritvo PG, Siu SC, Webb GD. Prevalence and correlates of successful transfer from pediatric to adult health care among a cohort of young adults with complex congenital heart defects. Pediatrics 2004;113(3):e197-205..

[13] Shaw KL, Southwood TR, McDonagh JE. Transitional care for adolescents with juvenile idiopathic arthritis: a Delphi study. Rheumatology 2004;43(8):1000-6..
[14] Boyle MP, Farukhi Z, Nosky ML. Strategies for improving transition to adult cystic fibrosis care, based on patient and parent views. Pediatr Pulmonol 2001; 32(6):428-36.
[15] Stabile L, Rosser L, Porterfiled KM, McCauley S, Levenson C, Haglund J, Christman K. Transfer versus transition: success in pediatric transplantation brings the welcome challenge of transition. Prog Transplant 2005;15(4):363-70.
[16] Reiss JG, Gibson RW, Walker LR. Health care transition: youth, family and provider perspectives. Pediatrics 2005;115(1):112-20.
[17] Tuchman LK, Slap GB, Britto ML. Transition to adult care: experiences and expectations of adolescents with a chronic illness. Child Care Health Dev 2008; 34(5):557-63.
[18] Anthony SJ, Kaufman M, Drabble A, Seifert-Hansen M, Dipchand AI, Martin K. Perceptions of transitional care needs and experiences in pediatric heart transplant Recipients. Am J Transplant 2009;9(3):614-9.

In: School, Adolescence and Health Issues
Editors: J. Merrick, A. Tenenbaum and H. A. Omar
ISBN: 978-1-62948-702-1

Chapter 11

ADOLESCENT BEREAVEMENT

Leslie Robin and Hatim A Omar, MD*

Division of Adolescent Medicine, Department of Pediatrics, University of Kentucky, Lexington, Kentucky, US

ABSTRACT

Depending on cognitive and emotional development, an adolescent may grieve very differently than a child or an adult. While mature enough to understand death's irreversibility, adolescents may not fully comprehend the enduring consequences of a loved one's death. As the desire to separate from their families and forge new intimate relationships with peers assumes increasing priority, adolescents can seem egocentric in their reaction to death, a response which often frustrates and perplexes adults. Because volatile behavior is characteristic of adolescence, health providers struggle to differentiate between normal and complicated bereavement. Here we review the commonly-accepted characteristics of normal and complicated grief for both early and middle adolescents and consider factors which influence adolescent bereavement, such as the relationship with the deceased, the circumstances of the death, and religious and cultural implications.

INTRODUCTION

Bereavement can be said to "encompass the entire experience of family members and friends in the anticipation, death and subsequent adjustment to living following the death of a loved one" (1). While much has been published regarding adult and child bereavement, however, there exists relatively little information regarding the bereavement of adolescents.

There is disagreement over what exactly constitutes normal adult bereavement, but at least three fundamental "tasks" have been identified: acknowledging the death, working through the pain, and finally accommodating the death (2).

* Correspondence: Professor Hatim A Omar, MD, J422 Kentucky Clinic, University of Kentucky, Lexington, KY 40536-0284, United States. E-mail: hatim.omar@uky.edu.

Acknowledging the death involves coming to terms with the circumstances and irreversibility of the death, a task which is relatively straightforward for adults, who possess the cognitive abilities to understand the causes and nature of death. Working through the pain is characterized by emotions such as sadness, anger, guilt, anxiety, helplessness, yearning, emancipation, and numbness, as well as physical symptoms such as chest tightness, stomach hollowness, heightened sensitivity to noise, shortness of breath, weakness, fatigue and dry mouth (3). During this phase the bereaved may also experience altered thought patterns such as disbelief, confusion, forgetfulness, decreased concentration, preoccupation, depersonalization, or even hallucinations in addition to behavioral changes like sleep disturbances, appetite changes, withdrawal, restlessness, and crying (3). Finally, the task of accommodating the death is marked by task reassignment (both day-to-day and emotional), redefinition of self, and ultimately the resumption of life cycle tasks (3). This task is also known as reconstitution, which when successful "results in decrease in the frequency and intensity of grief and a gradual return to previous levels of functioning"(4). Most adults accomplish reconstitution within 6 – 12 months of a loved one's death.

Bereavement in Adolescence

The death of a loved one takes a considerable emotional toll on normally-functioning adults, but the effects are typically more pronounced in adolescents, as "coping with death and grief is not a normative life transition for an adolescent" (5). While children and adolescents must progress through the same bereavement tasks as adults, their unique psychological defenses and cognitive and emotional development affect their expression of grief (3).

In general, children and adolescents experience the intense emotions of bereavement in shorter episodes than adults, punctuated by periods during which they resume normal activities (4). Because they are still developing, they may struggle with the already cyclical nature of grief more than adults as "each new developmental step requires children to reinterpret the death" based on new cognitive or emotional understandings (3). Thus the grieving process may appear shorter for adolescents, but may actually reoccur via reinterpretations until adulthood.

Early Adolescence (12-14 years): During this developmental period, teens experience pubertal physiological changes which may cause marked mood swings and sometimes explosive displays of emotion as hormones surge. Egocentric behavior is common as early adolescents begin to withdraw emotionally from their families in an effort to establish independence; at this stage, however, most teens are conflicted between desiring independence but still being very much dependent on their caretakers emotionally and otherwise. Formal operational thinking in early adolescents is inconsistent, and the preferred psychological defense mechanisms may include regression, denial, and self-limiting exposure to overwhelming emotions (3, 4). Most notably, peer acceptance assumes apical priority during early adolescence (6, 7).

As a result of these developmental features, early adolescents grieve differently than adults. The behaviors characterizing normal bereavement depend not only on the circumstances of the loss but also the adolescent's preexisting developmental stage. In acknowledging the death, most early adolescents are able to comprehend its irreversibility and causes in a manner similar to adults, but may be disinterested in the specific details surrounding the death, especially if it is the result of a long-term illness (7). Early adolescents' reactions to death can often seem selfish or egocentric, as they may be more concerned with the impact that the death will have on them than about the deceased or family members (8).

The task of working through the pain is typically quite different for early adolescents than for adults. Due to the paramount importance placed on social acceptance, young teens are often reluctant to express their emotions in front of peers (4); the perceived inability to grieve in public may cause them to behave callously toward the illness or needs of a family member, especially if there is a negative stigma associated with the death (9). In an effort to maintain a degree of independence from their families, they may wish to grieve privately and avoid family discussions, but the intense emotions associated with adult grief may surface in explosive bursts (4).

Complicated bereavement in early adolescents is characterized by school refusal, persistent anhedonia or depression, initiation of drug or alcohol use, shoplifting, shifting to a more delinquent group of friends, or precocious sexual behavior; their behavior may become oppositional, argumentative, and demanding (4). Young adolescents experiencing complicated bereavement may also make somatic complaints with no obvious etiology (4). These symptoms should be evaluated within the context of the young adolescent's behavior and psychological countenance prior to the death, however, to determine if they are actually indicative of complicated bereavement.

Middle Adolescence (15-17 years): Depending on the emotional maturity of the middle adolescent, he or she may exhibit many of the characteristics of early adolescent bereavement. Often, however, middle adolescents "are more constrained in their behavior, more understanding of situational demands, and, although they remain resentful, often exhibit more empathy concerning [other peoples'] needs than early adolescents"(4). Because they are better able to comprehend the enduring consequences of death, middle adolescents acknowledge death in a manner very similar to adults in that they are able to confront death more directly before it occurs if possible and to better appreciate future consequences (4).

The way in which a middle adolescent works through the pain of grief depends largely on his or her stage of emotional and cognitive development prior to the loss. The typical middle adolescent uses formal operational development more consistently and demonstrates integration of the future with the present and past (4). Older teens are generally more thoughtful, allocentric, and empathetic than early adolescents, but still struggle to balance the needs of others with their own egocentric desires (4). By middle adolescence, males tend to separate from their parents, while girls tend to alter their relationships with their parents (4).

During normal bereavement middle adolescents experience overwhelming sadness and painful memories like adults, but for a shorter duration. If the adolescent's family is also bereaved, he or she may be easily overwhelmed by or intolerant of their emotional dependence (4). Continuing to establish their independence, most middle adolescents have formed intimate supportive relationships with peers which can sometimes be helpful in working through the pain of bereavement. In the event that these friends misunderstand the bereaved's grief or even reject him or her for it, however, the adolescent may be devastated and grieve not only the death of a loved one, but the loss of a cherished extrafamilial relationship (10).

All adolescents: While each teen grieves uniquely, a clear indication of complicated bereavement is the inability to resume normal cognitive and emotional development (11-13). While the time required for reconstitution varies among individuals, "studies suggest that by 6 to 12 months, most adolescents are well on the road to accomplishing [successful reconstitution]" (11, 14, 15). For both early and middle adolescents, the task of accommodating the death, or reconstitution, involves not only mourning the loss of the deceased and forming new relationships with the deceased and survivors, but overcoming barriers to fulfilling developmental tasks.

If the death occurred within the adolescent's family, he or she may suffer a lack of confidence in independent functioning or feel hindered in his or her emotional withdrawal from the family (4). In acknowledging the death, middle adolescents may fear that they are unable to handle future independence and may become concerned about their own mortality, especially if a family member died as a result of illness (4).

Adolescents' peer acceptance and the emergence of intimacy with peers are other developmental tasks challenged by the death of a loved one. Adolescents typically fear strong emotions, and as such may abandon the bereaved adolescent, especially if he or she displays signs of emotional distress (10, 16). With such a tremendous importance placed on social acceptance and peer relationships, such a rejection can compound a teen's preexisting grief, complicating and prolonging the bereavement process.

Accommodating the death, characterized by a redefinition of self in adults, is further complicated by the fact that early adolescents do not typically enter the bereavement process with a strong sense of self (3, 5). Not surprisingly, the more trouble an adolescents have with self-definition and coping prior to the death, the more vulnerable they are to complicated bereavement.

Complicated bereavement

While there is significant debate as to what constitutes complicates bereavement, there are eight indicative symptoms: "longing and searching for the deceased, preoccupation with thoughts of the deceased, purposelessness and futility about the future, numbness and detachment from others, difficulty accepting the death, lost sense of security and control, and anger and bitterness over the death"(17). To fulfill diagnosis the bereaved must experience at least four of these symptoms for at least six months, and have experienced "considerable impairment in social, occupational, and other major areas of functioning"(9). Complicated grief has been linked to functional impairment, even after controlling for depression, anxiety, and posttraumatic stress disorder (17).

Put simply, complicated bereavement is chronic grief which precludes the resumption of normal life functions; people exhibiting complicated grief are significantly derailed by a death and fail to "move on." In adolescents, bereavement is considered complicated when it significantly hinders a teen's cognitive and social development into an adult. Between 13% and 17% of bereaved children and adolescents are reported to exhibit this ineffective reconstitution (12, 14, 18, 19).

Despite these definitions of "normal" and "complicated" grief, it must be noted that every person grieves uniquely, and that many factors influence the grieving process (20). The characteristics of the bereaved individual and the availability of support must be evaluated on an individual basis; low self-esteem, preexisting mental health problems, and a negative or non-supportive relationship with caregivers are certainly factors which increase one's risk of experiencing complicated bereavement (4).

The grieving process also depends significantly on the circumstances of the death, the bereaved's relationship with the deceased, and myriad sociocultural factors.

Homicide

When compared to all other types of death, violent homicide is associated with the most complicated grief (21). Not surprisingly, the risk of complicated grief is higher when the death is sudden, unexpected, and/or violent (9). Homicide survivors must confront both grief and trauma simultaneously, and therefore are particularly susceptible to posttraumatic stress disorder (22). When a death could have been prevented, such as in the case of homicide, the grieving process can be complicated by survivor anger, a lack of closure, feelings of victimization, obsession and rumination, a search for meaning, and the need to assign blame or mete out punishment (23). In their quest for independence, adolescents often experience conflict with their loved ones and may feel intense guilt about these arguments if loved one is killed.

The most significant complication that adolescents experience after the homicidal death is an altered worldview; adolescence is the time during which individuals develop moral reasoning and an understanding of the consequences of their actions, and grieving a homicide can undermine this process (24). Homicide can confound adolescents' understanding of societal norms, their sense of right and wrong, and even their respect for human life (25). This disruption in normal development is often compounded by a lack of social support due to the negative stigma associated with death by homicide, causing the adolescent's complicated bereavement to be even more pronounced (23). Overall, the more violent the crime and the more directly it is witnessed by the bereaved, the more likely he or she is to experience complicated bereavement (26).

Suicide

Adolescents bereaved by suicide are at risk for many of the same complications as those bereaved by homicide, but the negative stigma associated with suicide poses an even greater threat to their normal social development; people bereaved by suicide are at a greater risk of experiencing stigmatization, shame, guilt, and a sense of rejection than those bereaved by other causes of death (27). Adolescents often grieve in isolation, experiencing a lack of social support and a personal sense of ineffectiveness (28). This social isolation, in conjunction with the mood disorders commonly associated with bereavement, sometimes begets suicidal ideation or behavior, although actual suicide attempts are rare (29). Depression, anxiety, and posttraumatic stress are the most prevalent complications experienced by adolescents grieving a suicide death especially within the first 6 to 12 months (28, 30). When an adolescent is bereaved by the suicide of a family member the risk is greater due to the potential emotional unavailability of parents and relatives who are grieving themselves; parental psychopathology and stressful life circumstances have been shown to exacerbate psychiatric symptoms and poor social adjustment (28).

WARS, TERRORISM, DISASTER AND OTHER SUDDEN DEATHS

Those bereaved by sudden death are more likely to experience a sense of unreality, of helplessness, heightened feelings of guilt for failing to prevent the death, and a strong need to blame someone for the death, much like those bereaved by homicide and suicide (31). Often the pain and shock following a sudden death are so overwhelming that the bereaved is simply incapable of grieving, and the process gets postponed; sometimes the resolution of legal or medical issues provides the closure necessary to grieve (32, 33).

Children and adolescents exposed to war are particularly prone to posttraumatic stress, with the severity typically depending on the extent to which sudden death is witnessed, although the cumulative exposure, intensity, and duration of the exposure have been suggested to be more impacting than the specific events witnessed (34). The prevalence of posttraumatic stress among children exposed to war varies from 10 to 90%, manifested by disorders such as PTSD, depression, disruptive behaviors, and somatic symptoms, with females more inclined to manifest anxiety symptoms and males exhibiting more disruptive behavior (34, 35). When sudden death affects many people at once, such as in the case of terrorist attacks or school shootings, solidarity among survivors can be a positive influence in that it helps to make a bizarre event seem more normal and universal; the burden of grief is shared especially by those who realize that they could just as easily have been killed (33). When survivors of war share a strong sense of group identification, shared values, common values and social cohesiveness, their grief is less likely to be complicated (34).

LONG-TERM ILLNESS

Although there is little data reporting adolescents' bereavement following the terminal illness of a loved one, children and adolescents typically exhibit more symptoms of depression, anxiety, and lower self-esteem during the terminal illness than they do after the death (15). When adolescents whose parents have survived cancer are compared with those whose parents were killed by the disease, there was no significant difference in their anxiety and stress; when compared to adults in comparable bereavement situations, however, adolescents were found to exhibit more anxiety and depressions symptoms than adults (36). This is consistent with the findings for adults; it has been suggested that the more strain experienced by the caregiver before death, the less likely the caregiver to report increased symptoms of depression after the death (37, 38).

One factor which increased the likelihood of experiencing complicated grief was a perceived lack of preparedness for the death (39). Depending on the severity and conditions of the terminal illness, the adolescent may even feel relieved after the death, having dealt with depression and familial stress throughout the illness.

PARENTAL DEATH

Five percent of children in the US will lose a parent by the age of 16 years (3). The death of a parent during adolescence can be especially difficult to cope with. Parents typically function as safe, supportive figures who sustain, regulate affect, and repair aspects of the self (40). Without this support adolescents may struggle with the formative process developing a strong sense of self. On the other hand, adolescence is the period during which teens break bonds with their parents and establish their independence, a process to which parental loss is conducive. Thus there is an intertwining of two grief experiences: a normative developmental desire for independence, and the non-normative response to death (41).

When compared to adults who are parentally bereaved, adolescents display more intense grief reactions and more negative interpersonal perceptions, as well as more sleep problems, irritability, anger, feelings of emptiness, and difficulty interacting with others (42). Parentally bereaved adolescents also reported more concerns about fairness surrounding death, and intense, personal sense of loss, feelings that the deceased parent is irreplaceable, and a strong presence of the deceased in dreams and other people (43). They may identify with specific ambitions or goals shared with the parent whose life ended prematurely, leading to an exacerbation of the grieving process (44). The most significant difference between parentally bereaved adolescents and adults is that adolescents seem to suffer more social and interpersonal difficulties; they tend to feel isolated and exhibit a strong desire for others to include them and take interest in them (43). This is probably because it is much more common and socially acceptable for adults to lose parents.

Also exacerbating the grieving process for parentally bereaved adolescents is the fact that a parental death almost always involves the destabilization of the family structure. Often the adolescent must adjust to new guardianship, whether it be the surviving parent or other relatives. It is also common for the surviving parent to at least initially be overly dependent or emotionally needy, something adolescents may resent (44).

SIBLING DEATH

It is estimated that siblings spend 80-100% of their lives together, more time than with any other family member (45); marriages often end in divorce and family structures may dissolve, but siblings are almost always kept together. Because of this shared history, siblings are intricately connected such that when a sibling dies the survivors essentially lose a part of themselves (46).

Siblings play a crucial role in identity development, a process which is of particular importance during adolescence. After the death, bereaved siblings tend to examine their lives and maintain bonds with the deceased not only by treasuring his or her memory, but also by continuing the relationship; many bereaved adolescents report feeling like their deceased siblings are "still with them" or are "watching over them" (47). Bereaved siblings often maintain connections with their deceased brother or sister by cherishing favorite mementos and pictures, and even having ongoing conversations (48). This continuing relationship is renegotiated as the surviving sibling reaches new developmental stages or life milestones (46).

The way in which an adolescent is affected by the death of a sibling depends largely on the family dynamics before and after the death. If the sibling relationship was warm and caring, the continuing bonds with the deceased sibling are expected to be positive and comforting, whereas a hostile or adversarial sibling relationship will likely yield continuing bonds which are disturbing (49). Likewise, the closer and more united the family is prior to the death, the less likely the adolescent is to experience complicated bereavement (50).

Sibling loss is often referred to as a double loss, because the bereaved not only loses a brother or sister, but also their parents' support; in grieving their deceased children, many parents simply lack the emotional energy to adequately care for their surviving children (48). People often fail to appreciate the extent to which sibling survivors suffer, instead focusing on their parents' grief, urging teens to "remain strong for their parents" (46). If parents are preoccupied with the immortalization of the deceased child, surviving children feel neglected and less important, whereas if parents are avoidant and make no references to the deceased child then the surviving children feel forced to grieve alone (48).

Surviving children sometimes feel intense guilt, especially if their sibling's death was the result of an accident in which they were involved (8). They may also feel disloyal in moving on with their lives and leaving their deceased sibling behind (46). In addition to grief, surviving siblings may experience feelings of isolation and inadequacy, especially if their parents seem inconsolable.

Parents may feel incompetent or guilty over the child's death, and as such may become hypervigilant or overprotective of surviving child, causing additional tension (8).

FRIEND OR PEER DEATH

Peers play a central role in the development of an adolescent's identity and self-esteem, and as such the loss of a friend can be devastating. Unlike the death of grandparents or other family members, adolescent deaths are much more likely to be sudden and unexpected, and adolescents usually learn of the death from other peers as opposed to their parents or doctors (51, 52).

A common sentiment reported by teens who have lost peers is that the peer was too young to have died (53). The death of a peer forces adolescents to confront the issue of their own mortality, an unsettling and destabilizing process for adolescents who otherwise tend to feel invincible (53). In this context ambitions and idealism can seen futile, even absurd, as grieving adolescents are enveloped by a pervasive sense of purposelessness (53). Although reports of suicidal ideation are common, especially immediately after the death, suicide attempts and completions rarely result (27). If the peer died as a result of suicide, however, the likelihood of significant depression and fascination with dramatic, sensational, or romantic death among adolescent survivors is much greater, and cluster suicides may occur (8, 54).

Three factors dictate how an adolescent is affected by the death of a peer: the importance of that peer to the adolescent's self-esteem, the role of the peer in the adolescent's identity formation, and the extent to which that peer assumed many of the protective emotional functions originally performed by the adolescent's parents (53). Adults often fail to realize the critical importance of peer relationships to adolescent development, and may be dismissive about the extent of their grief. This is especially pronounced if the deceased was a role model or significant other to the bereaved (55). By minimizing the significance of peer relationships adults can complicate the adolescent's already painful grief.

CULTURAL CONSIDERATIONS

When seeking to understand an adolescent's grief as complicated or not, one must also consider his or her cultural or religious background.

There are many things to consider: the traditions and rituals for coping with dying, the deceased's body, and honoring the deceased, the beliefs about what happens after death, the characteristics of a normal expression of grief, the roles of family members in coping with death, and whether there are certain types of death which may be less acceptable or especially hard to handle (56). Teens have been shown to become more religious following the death of a loved one since (47, 57):

- Emerging cognitive abilities allow adolescent to consider religious beliefs in new ways
- Adolescence is the time when religious values and beliefs can be clarified
- They may be able to construct an image of God in new ways
- Organized religion is often structured in a way that provides support and encourages coping
- Religion gives meaning to many situations and can signify a sense of control, growth, hope, intimacy
- Provides meanings to release and redemption
- Death can be viewed as a release from burden, pain, and the relationship to suffering
- Death may mean redemption as it can signify freedom from what binds us to earth and can eventually lead to a reunion with loved ones

DISCUSSION

There exists an inherent paradox in the wealth of grief and bereavement literature. On the one hand, there is an understandable effort to define what, exactly, constitutes "normal" versus "complicated" bereavement so that health professionals may refer to some objective diagnostic protocol when deciding whether a patient's bereavement warrants intervention. On the other hand, it is widely acknowledged that every person grieves differently. How, then, can physicians or parents determine when intervention is necessary to treat complicated grief? The broad answer to this question is that, although bereavement is not a normative life function for adolescents, it should not significantly interrupt their normal cognitive and emotional development. In order to know when an adolescent's development has been effectively derailed, however, physicians cannot simply consult developmental benchmarks; rather they must consider the teen's grief holistically, taking into account the many variables which influence bereavement, including the circumstances of the death, the relationship between the adolescent and the deceased, and the emotional support available to the adolescent.

The better acquainted a physician is with the adolescent prior to the bereavement experience, the easier it will be for him or her to diagnose complicated grief. Without the benefit of baseline assessment, physicians must rely heavily upon circumstantial clues to understand their adolescent patients' bereavement. Even without the benefit of prior exposure, however, physicians should approach grieving adolescents from a developmental perspective, taking into account their available coping mechanisms at the time of death.

Unlike adults, whose reconstitution essentially involves resuming the life activities which predated the death, adolescents do struggle with developing a strong sense of self while simultaneously grieving the loss of a loved one. Bereavement is not a normal adolescent developmental task, and as such it seems likely to influence a teen's self-definition. This is not necessarily a negative influence; many adolescents emerge stronger, more mature, and more tolerant of others' emotions after bereavement. The extent to which bereavement influences adolescents' development for better or for worse, however, depends largely on their maturity and coping strategies prior to the death and the support they receive while grieving. Thus for the sake of patients' proper maturation into adults, physicians treating bereaved adolescents must take a proactive role in the bereavement process to assure they have access to necessary services and support.

References

[1] Christ G, Bonanno G, Malkinson R, Rubin S. Bereavement experiences after the death of a child. In: Field M, Behrman R, eds. When children die: Improving palliative care for children and their families. Washington, DC: Natl Acad Press, 2003:554.

[2] Worden JW. Grief counseling and grief therapy. A handbook for the mental health practitioner, 2nd ed. New York: Springer, 1991.

[3] Schultz K. Bereaved children. Can Fam Physician 1999;45:2914-21.

[4] Christ H, Siegel K, Christ A. Adolescent grief: "it never really hit me…until it actually happened." JAMA 2002;288:1269-78.

[5] Balk D. Models for understanding adolescent coping with bereavement. Death Stud 1996;20:367-87.

[6] Blos P. On adolescence. New York: Macmillan, 1962.

[7] Christ G. Impact of development on children's mourning. Cancer Pract 2000;8:72-81.

[8] Serwint J. Chapter 17. Separation, loss, and bereavement. In: Kleigman R, Behrman R, Jenson H, Stranton B, eds. Nelson textbook of pediatrics, 18th ed. Philadelphia, PA. Saunders Elsevier, 2007.

[9] Hawton K. Complicated grief after bereavement. Psychological interventions may be effective. BMJ 2007;334:962-3.

[10] Gray R. Adolescents' perceptions of social support after the death of a parent. J Psychosoc Oncol 1989;7:127-44.

[11] Worden J. Children and grief: when a parent dies. New York: Guilford, 1996.

[12] Christ G. Healing children's grief: surviving a parent's death from cancer. New York: Oxford Univ Press, 2000.

[13] Silverman P, Nickman S, Worden J. Detachment revisited. In: Doka K, ed. Children's mourning, mourning in children. Washington, DC: Hospice Foundation of America, 1995:131-48.

[14] Siegel K, Raveis V, Karus D. Patterns of communication with children when a parent has cancer. In: Baider L, Cooper C, De Nour A, eds. Cancer and the family. New York: John Wiley, 1996:109-28.

[15] Siegel K, Karus D, Raveis VH. Adjustment of children facing the death of a parent due to cancer. J Am Acad Adolesc Psychiatry 1996;35:442-50.

[16] Tyson-Rawson K. Adolescent responses to the death of a parent. In: Corr C, Balk D, eds. Handbook of adolescent death and bereavement. New York: Springer, 1996:155-72.

[17] Melhem N, Moritz G, Walker M, Shear M, Brent D. Phenomenology and correlates of complicated grief in children and adolescents. J Am Acad Child Adolesc Psychiatry 2007;46(4):493-9.

[18] Siegel K, Mesagno R, Christ G. A preventative program for bereaved children. Am J Orthopsychiatry 1990;60:168-75.

[19] Saltzman W, Pynoos R, Layne C. Trauma/grief focused intervention for adolescents exposed to community violence: results of school-based screening and group treatment protocol. Group Dynamics Theory Res Pract 2001;5:291-303.

[20] Breen LJ, O'Connor M. The fundamental paradox in the grief literature: a critical reflection. Omega 2007;55(3):199-218.

[21] Cable DG. Grief counseling for survivors of traumatic loss. In: Doka K, ed. Living with grief after sudden loss: Suicide, homicide, accident, heart attack, stroke. Washington, DC: Hospice Foundation of America, 2007:117-26.

[22] Clements P, Burgess AW. Children's responses to family member homicide. Fam Community Health 2002;25(1):32-42.

[23] Vigil G, Clements P. Child and adolescent homicide survivors. Complicated grief and altered worldviews. J Psychosoc Nurs Ment Health Serv 2003;41(1):30-9.

[24] Pynoos RS, Nader K. Issues in the treatment of posttraumatic stress in children and adolescents. International handbook of traumatic stress syndromes. New York: Plenum, 1993.

[25] Burgess AW, Hartman C, Clements P. The biology of memory in childhood trauma. Journal of psychosocial Nurs Ment Health Serv 1995;33(3):16-26.

[26] Clements P, Weisser S. Cries from the morgue. J Child Adolesc Psychiatr Nurs 2003;16(4):153-61.

[27] Jordan JR. Is suicide bereavement different? A reassessment of the literature. Suicide Life Threat Behav 2006;31:91-102.

[28] Pfeffer C, Martins P, Mann JJ, Sunkenberg M, Ice A, Damore J, et al. Child survivors of suicide: psychosocial characteristics. J Am Acad Child Adolesc Psychiatry 1997;36(1):65-74.

[29] Pfeffer CR. The suicidal child. New York: Guilford, 1986.

[30] Brent DA, Perper JA, Moritz G, et al. Psychiatric impact of the loss of an adolescent sibling to suicide. J Affect Disord 1993;28:249-56.

[31] Rynearson EK. Bereavement after homicide: a descriptive study. Am J Psychiatry 1984;141:1452-4.

[32] Fulton R, Gottesman DJ. Anticipatory grief: a psychosocial concept to be reconsidered. Br J Psychiatry 1980;137:45-54.

[33] Fast J. After Columbine: How people mourn sudden death. Soc Work 2003;48(4):484-92.

[34] Shaw JA. Children exposed to was/terrorism. Clin Child Fam Psychol Rev 2003;6(4):237-46.

[35] Allwood MA, Bell-Dolan D, Husain SA. Children's trauma and adjustment reactions to violent and nonviolent war experiences. JAm Acad Child Adolesc Psychiatry 2002;41:450-7.

[36] Mireault GC, Compas BE. A prospective study of coping and adjustment before and after a parent's death from cancer. J Psychosoc Oncol 1996;14:1-18.

[37] Shulz R, Beach S, Lind B, Martire L, Zdaniuk B, Hirsch C, Jackson S, Burton L. Involvement in caregiving and adjustment to death of a spouse: findings from the caregiver health effects study. JAMA 2001;285:3123-9.

[38] Chentsova-Dutton Y, Schucter S, Hutchin S, Strause L, Burns K, Dunn L, et al. Depression and grief reactions in hospice caregivers: from pre-death to 1 year afterwards. J Affect Disord 2002;69:53-60.

[39] Barry L, Kasl S, Prigerson H. Psychiatric disorders among bereaved persons: the role of perceived circumstances of death and preparedness for death. Am J Geriatr Psychiatry 2002;10:447-57.

[40] Sussillo M. Beyond the grave—adolescent parental loss. Letting go and holding on. Psychoanal Dialogues 2005;15(4):499-527.

[41] Garber B. Mourning in adolescence: normal and pathological. Ann Am Society Adolesc Psychiatry 1985;16:511-25.

[42] Servaty-Seib H, Hayslip B. Post-loss adjustment and funeral perceptions of parentally bereaved adolescents and adults. Omega 2002-2003;46(3):251-61.

[43] Meshot CM, Leitner LM. Adolescents' mourning and parental death. Omega 1993;26:287-99.

[44] Tyson-Rawson KJ. Adolescent responses to the death of a parent. In: Corr CA, Balk DE eds. Handbook of adolescent death and bereavement. New York: Springer, 1996:155-72.
[45] Bank SP, Kahn MD. The sibling bond. New York: Basic Books, 1982.
[46] Devita-Raeburn E. The empty room: surviving the loss of a brother or sister at any age. New York: Scribner 2004.
[47] Batten M, Oltjenbruns KA. Adolescent sibling bereavement as a catalyst for spiritual development: a model for understanding. Death Stud 1999;23:529-46.
[48] Packman W, Horsley H, Davies B, Kramer R. Sibling bereavement and continuing bonds. Death Stud 2006;30:817-41.
[49] Normand CL, Silverman PR, Nickman SL. Bereaved children's changing relationship with the deceased. In: Silverman PR, Nickman SL eds. Continuing bonds: new understandings of grief. Philadelphia, PA: Taylor Francis 1996:87-111.
[50] Davies B. Toward siblings' understanding and perspective of death. In: Grollman E, ed. Bereaved children and teens: a support guide for parents and professionals. Boston, MA: Beacon Press, 1995:61-74.
[51] Ringler L, Hayden D. Adolescent bereavement and social support: peer loss compared to other losses. J Adolesc Res 2000;15:209-30.
[52] Report on Bereavement and Grief Research. Death Stud 2004;28(6):491-575.
[53] Podell S. Suicide intervention in the schools. New York: Guilford, 1989.
[54] Brent D, Perper J, Moritz G, Allman C, Liotus L, Schweers J, et al. Bereavement of depression? The impact of the loss of a friend to suicide. J Am Acad Child Adolesc Psychiatry 1993;32(6):1189-97.
[55] Raphael B. The anatomy of bereavement. New York: Basic Books, 1983:167-8.
[56] Clements PT, Vigil GJ, Manno MS, Henry G, Wilks J, Das S, et al. Cultural perspectives of death, grief, and bereavement. J Psychosoc Nurs 2003;41(7):18-26.
[57] Balk DE. Death and adolescent bereavement. J Adolesc Res 1991;6:7-27.

In: School, Adolescence and Health Issues
Editors: J. Merrick, A. Tenenbaum and H. A. Omar
ISBN: 978-1-62948-702-1

Chapter 12

THEATRICAL GAMES: SCHOOLCHILDREN AND FAMILIARISATION WITH THE MEANING OF LOSS AND DEATH

Angeliki Nikolakopoulou, BSc, PhD, Fotini Garagouni–Areou, BSc, PhD, Christina Roussi-Vergou, BSc, PhD and Maria Zafiropoulou, BSc, PhD*

Laboratory of Developmental Psychology and Psychopathology,
Department of Preschool Education, University of Thessaly,
Volos, Greece

ABSTRACT

Death and loss are undoubtedly some of the most emotionally painful events in a child's life. The research questions dealt with in this chapter are a) whether familiarisation with loss and death differs between children from urban and rural regions and b) whether theatrical games dealing with loss of a loved one could facilitate familiarisation with the meaning of death. One hundred and ninety one 3rd grade school students from Greek urban and rural regions participated in the study. Children were divided in four groups (2 experimental and 2 control groups).

Children in the experimental groups participated in a theatrical game with death as a subject, while control groups engaged themselves with artistic and sports activities. All participants were appropriately interviewed before and after the intervention. According to results children's knowledge and familiarisation with death improved after implementation of the theatrical game.

* Correspondence: Professor Maria Zafiropoulou, PhD, Department of Pre-School Education, University of Thessaly, Argonafton and Filellinon Street, Volos 38221, Greece. E-mail: mzafirop@ece.uth.gr.

INTRODUCTION

Death is a matter of grievous concern for children of all ages, except for those in very early childhood. It fills them with numerous questions about its nature and effects, and often causes them awe and fear. Relative literature describes death as the hidden cause of any pain (1), or as most predictable, though sad and unexpected (2). Usually, looking for answers about death emerges during the stormy years of adolescence (2).

The way each child perceives death depends on their cognitive, emotional and physical developmental stage. The three main aspects of death, namely universality, irreversibility and non-functionality, are understood as children grow older. Speece and Brent (3) in their in-depth literature review found many differences among researchers dealing with this issue. However, they concluded that, by the age of 7, most children have come to understand the above mentioned three concepts.

According to many researchers, learning about loss, death and lament can help students prepare themselves to actually face such an experience. They can also understand that grief is normal, and therefore they are not out of their minds, when grieving. Furthermore, learning about death and loss helps children understand the feelings of other classmates who experience the death of a loved one or other significant losses and can sympathize with them. (4). Moreover, emotional development during childhood enables children to understand the complexity of emotions and to show empathy for others' feelings (5, 6), while they show volatility of their emotions (7).

Theatrical games increase children's ability to communicate, since they see and are being seen, listen and answer, understand and are being understood, and all these are accomplished on many different levels, depending on the topics selected, each time (8).

Theatrical games, in the context of applied psychology, give children the opportunity for externalisation of thoughts and emotions. At the same time, drama acts as a regulator of any emotional burden, tension, aggression, etc. A theatrical game relaxes, releases children's creativity and facilitates internal balance (9).

Two tragic road accidents which affected the whole of the Greek school community and caused extreme, but justifiable, psychological shock, launched the present study. Moreover, the awkwardness that teachers of all grades feel when they face such problems within school communities show that dealing with death in a way which indicates deliberate ignorance or even aversion should be seriously reconsidered within education.

There is a special protocol with guidelines for teachers and headmasters on how to manage death in school and to deal with such events. This protocol has been adopted by the U.S., Canada and many European countries (10), but not by Greece. A research study conducted nationally by the University of Athens, in which 1792 teachers participated, revealed that Greek schools have no organized intervention programs which could provide appropriate guidance to support a grieving student (11). Although school psychologists could provide assistance in this area, yet, such an institution does not exist within Greek schools unlike other European countries. It appears, therefore, that integration of the concepts of loss and death in the school curriculum is sine qua non. It is essential that students familiarize themselves with these concepts with the implementation of suitable psycho-educational techniques, depending on their age level. In this chapter we want to:

- record elementary school children's level of knowledge, familiarity, and attitude towards the concept of death, in relation to their origin (urban or rural environment)
- determine whether the above-mentioned parameters could alter after implementation of an appropriate intervention.

OUR SAMPLE

The sample consisted of 191 3rd grade students (147 students from urban and 44 from rural areas of Central Greece), who were divided into 4 research groups (2 experimental and 2 control groups) as follows:

- The urban sample was divided into two groups [Urban A (UA) and Urban B (UB)]. The students in UA participated in a theatrical game which referred to death. The students in UB, the control group, engaged themselves with artistic and sports activities and participated only in the initial interview.
- The rural sample was also divided into two groups [Rural A (RA) and Rural B (RB)]. As in the previous case, students in RA participated in a theatrical game dealing with death, while students in RB, the control group, engaged themselves with artistic and sports activities taking part only in the interview.

RESEARCH TOOLS

The following methodological tools were used for the purpose of the study:

- A questionnaire recording the health and social background of the participants was used, in order for children with emotional disorders, children suffering from malignant disease, those who had recently experienced loss or had seriously ill parents, etc. to be excluded from the study.
- A theatrical game dealing with the death of a loved one (an imaginary grandmother) was created especially for the purpose of the study.
- An interview was also especially designed for the purpose of the study. The questions posed to the children were grouped so as to examine: a) children's perception of death, and b) level of their knowledge and familiarity with the concept of death.

More specifically,

- *Children's perception* was examined with questions based on the three main parameters of the death concept which, according to Childers & Wimmer (12), Beauchamp (13) and Speece & Brent (3), are universality, irreversibility and non-functionality. (i.e., "Do you think death of an individual is temporary or permanent?", or "Do all people die?" etc.).

- *Children's knowledge of death* was examined with questions concerning knowledge of the rituals of death (i.e., "Can you mention some customs that take place during a funeral?") and, finally,
- *Children's familiarity with death* was examined with questions related to children's experiences with death and their attitudes towards death (i.e., "Have you ever attended a funeral?", "Would you like to hear a story that refers to death?").

Process

The research process consisted of three sessions. During the first meeting the researcher met the students, drew their consent to participate in the study, and, finally, recorded information regarding their health and social background. During the second meeting students in both experimental groups participated in the theatrical game, whilst students in both control groups spent their time (the same length of time as the experimental groups) engaging with activities such as painting, free play and sports in the company of the researcher. Finally, the interviews were conducted.

The theatrical game referred to the death of an imaginary grandmother and was developed in the following stages:

Stage A: Liberation and acquaintance

Participants made a circle and were instructed to release themselves from any inhibitions. Each child said its name and interests.

In the middle of the circle a chair was placed and on the top of that chair a shawl was placed symbolizing an old woman (the grandmother). Students were asked to identify the symbol (shawl) to the image of real granny and to get to know her.

Stage B: Role playing game

In this stage children chose and played roles, and improvised short dialogues. They described how they thought the features and character of the grandmother were, and, at the same time, their "experiences' with the imaginary grandmother were recorded. More precisely, each child mentioned a pleasant or an unpleasant experience s/he had with granny i.e., a story or an adventure they had in the park, at home, at sea, etc. Students also described how they spend their spare time with her, what games they play together, or what tales and stories she tells them.

Stage C: Stage improvisation

Once the scenic area was formed, the stage of development and implementation of the thematic axis (death) began. That is, the grandmother's symbol (shawl) leaves the chair, because granny was taken to hospital. Students were asked to say:

- How they were feeling about granny being ill.
- If they went to visit her in the hospital.
- What granny's illness is and if she will manage to live.
- What they would like to happen regarding the progress of granny's health.

Then the animator, who pretended to be a doctor, gave children little envelopes and asked that each child wrote a wish for granny.

When grandmother's death was announced to the children, they were asked to relax and stop thinking about the grandmother's hospitalisation.

Finally, each child was given a little envelope, where the following phrase was written: *"I did not leave you. I'm in heaven now and I will be watching you from up there ".*

Stage D: Analysis-discussion

Children were asked, once again, to make a circle. Each child was, then, given about 30 seconds to say goodbye to granny in its own way. Finally, a discussion took place and the theme of the theatrical game was analysed. Children expressed their views, emotions and concerns about granny's "journey". They also proposed solutions and displayed ideas.

FINDINGS

Statistical analyses were performed using SPSS 13.0, Chi-square (x^2) and Fisher's exact tests. As already mentioned, children's perception, knowledge and familiarization with death according to their origin (urban or rural) were investigated through interviews. Furthermore, the possibility of diversification in some of these parameters after the intervention was assessed. Comparisons among children in urban and rural areas were initially done and, then, the differences before and after the intervention were tested. Chi-square (x^2) two-sample test was used with our frequency data, with the following results.

Regarding children's perception, no differences were observed between children in the two communities. In fact, children in both groups were equally aware of the irreversibility of death.

On the other hand, in the case of knowledge and familiarity with death, results appeared to be statistically different. Namely, it was found that children in rural areas have significantly better knowledge and greater familiarity with the concept of death ($p < 0.005$). More precisely, children in rural areas knew most of the funeral rituals (x^2= 3,56, df= 1, p= 0,042), they reported attending more funeral ceremonies (x^2= 14,420, df= 1, $p < 0.001$) and, finally, a higher percentage of them would like to hear a story about death (x^2= 4,620, df= 1, p= 0,039).

A comparison was carried out among the above mentioned variables before and after intervention. The following findings came up: As far as perception is concerned, children seemed to have become more aware of the irreversibility of death after the intervention, but Fisher's exact test results did not show any statistically significant difference (x^2= 3,103, df= 1, p= 0,092). However, as far as familiarity is concerned, it was found that a greater number of children wanted to hear a story about death (x^2= 3,294, df= 1, p= 0,048).

DISCUSSION

According to the results of the present study, children from rural areas have better knowledge and exhibit greater familiarity with the concept of death. In an attempt to interpret this finding one could argue that in small communities, as those in rural areas, death is close to their daily lives (14). Children of rural origin seem to actually participate during the process and rituals of mourning. On the contrary, the lack of familiarity recorded in children from urban areas is consistent with almost all the literature referred to death. According to Benoliel (15), in the new urban environment, death and mortality are experiences and situations which take place more and more away from the average person. As a result, the separation of the dying from the living deprives youngsters from the social 'assistance' to familiarize themselves with the reality of death. Thus, a so-called society that declines death has been created (16). Taking care of the sick in the last stages of their life and making relevant decisions are no longer "a family issue", but it belongs to the experts, i.e., complex and impersonal settings such as hospitals, clinics, nursing homes, mainly in cities (17, 18). Young persons' lack of familiarity with death leads them to a situation where even the idea of their own death or death in general, fills them with great anxiety (14).

Special attention should also be given to the fact that familiarity with the concept of death was improved in the students of both communities, after the intervention. Similar results were demonstrated by an experimental method of teaching about familiarization and management of dying people, through dramatization followed by discussion, which was applied to first-year nurses, which seemed to work effectively in the education of nurses (19).

Therefore, the positive effect of expressing and experiencing emotions, negative ones in particular, through art is obvious. Yet, other kinds of art, apart from story telling and theatrical games, could be used so that the child is encouraged to "narrate" a powerful emotional experience. Drawing and painting are considered basic methods for either preventive or therapeutic intervention programs for children (20-22). As a result, many counselling psychology programs for children use drawing and painting as therapeutic means which serve many objectives (23, 24).

A particularly delicate issue is the one related to the methods that should be used in teaching about death. The subject of death should be treated with utmost sensitivity and be dealt with in a realistic and at the same time optimistic manner. Many researchers believe that learning about death should take place gradually through "small mourning" (25-27). The debate about death lies within small events or small deaths that occur in children's lives i.e., a dead bird found in the school yard, a tale that refers to the illness or death of the hero, etc. (28). The discussion about death could even start via art lessons, history, mathematics or science (29, 30).

In the light of the above findings, we believe that schools can play an important role in children's familiarization with the concept of death, by instructing students how to manage loss and grief experiences.

Finally, the present research study indicates that children's familiarity with the concept of loss is feasible and can occur in specific social contexts, where children have the opportunity to gain expertise and experiences. Yet, this indication certainly requires further investigation.

More specifically, it would be useful to further investigate whether the improved knowledge and familiarity observed after the intervention, are maintained over time with new interviews taken after two to six months in a follow-up process.

The familiarisation sessions should be more in number extending over a period of two-three months at least. This would allow for students' better understanding of the concept of death, through its three fundamental characteristics namely, universality, irreversibility and non-functionality. Finally, further attention should be given in the assessment of children's comprehension of the parameters of death. This is because the irreversibility and non-functionality of death might come into conflict with their already established religious beliefs, according to which soul is immortal.

REFERENCES

[1] Campbell J. The power of myth. London: Doubleday, 1988.
[2] Gersie A. And life goes on. Athens: Kedros, 2002. [Greek]
[3] Speece MN, Brent SB. Children's understanding of death: A Review of three components of death concept. Child Dev 1984;55:1671-86.
[4] Glass J, Conrad Jr. Death, loss, and grief among middle school children. Element Sch Guidance Couns 1991;26:139-48.
[5] Fabes R, Eisenberg N, Eisenbud L. Behavioural and psychological correlates of children's reactions to other in distress. Dev Psychol 1993;29:655-63.
[6] Strayer J. Children's concordant emotions and cognitions in response to observed emotions. Child Dev 1993;64:188–201.
[7] Zerman J. Emotional development. The Gale encyclopedia of childhood and adolescence. Detroit, MI: Gale Research, 1998.
[8] Faure G, Lascar S. The theatrical play. Athens: Gutenberg, 2001. [Greek].
[9] Kouretzis L. The theatrical play (Educational theory, practical and theatrological approach). Athens: Kastaniotis, 2001. [Greek]
[10] Stevenson RG, Powers HL. How to handle death in the school. Educ Digest 1987; 199-215.
[11] Papadatou D, Metallinou O, Xatzichristou C, Pavlidi L. Supporting the bereaved child: teacher's perception and experience in Greece. Mortality 2002;7(3):324-337.
[12] Childers P, Wimmer M. The concept of death in early childhood. Child Dev 1971; 42:1299-1301.
[13] Beauchamp NW. The young child's perception of death. (Doctoral dissertation Purdue University, 1974). Dissert Abstr Int 1974;35:3288A-3289A.
[14] Benoliel JQ, Denger LF. Institutional dying: A convergence of cultural values, technology, and social organization. In: Wass H, Neimeyer R, eds. Dying: Facing the facts, 3rd ed. Washington, DC: Taylor Francis, 1995:117-41.
[15] Benoliel JQ. Developments in thanatology. In: Nielsen M, Papadatou D, eds. Grief in our lives. Athens: Merimna, 1998:12-29. [Greek]
[16] Nielsen M, Papadatou D. Grief in our lives. Athens: Merimna, 1998 [Greek].
[17] Engel GL. The need for a new medical model: A challenge for Biomedicine. *Science* New Series 1977;196(4286):129-36.
[18] Møller DW. On dying without dignity: The human impact of technological dying. Amityville, NY: Baywood, 1990.
[19] Deeny P, Johnson A, Boore JRP, Leyden C, McCaughan EM. Drama as an experiential technique in learning how to cope with dying patients and their families. Teaching Higher Educ 2001;6(1):99-112.
[20] Barrett P, Wedser-Lowry H, Turner C. Friends for children workbook. Queensland: Australian Academic Press, 2000.
[21] Heegaard ME. Saying goodbye to your pet. Minneapolis, MN: Fairview Press, 2001.
[22] Stallard P. Think Good-Feel Good. Chichester: Wiley, 2002.
[23] Ronen T. Cognitive-developmental therapy with children. Chichester: Wiley, 1997.
[24] Geldard K, Geldard D. Counselling psychology with children. Theory-applications. Athens: Ellinika Grammata, 2004. [Greek]
[25] Kane B. Children's concepts of death. J Genet Psychol 1979;134:141-5.
[26] Stevenson RG. Death and school environment. In: Nielsen M, Papadatou D, eds. Grief in our lives. Athens: Merimna, 1998:97-106. [Greek]
[27] Bacque MF. Mourning and health then and now Athens: Thymari, 2001.[Greek]
[28] Papadatou D. The Child in front of illness and death. In: When sickness and death touched school life. Athens: Ministry of Education, 1999:15-25. [Greek]

[29] Stevenson RG. The role of the school to support children who are experiencing grief and mourning. In: Nielsen M, Papadatou D. When illness and death touched the school life Athens: Merimna, 1999:119-39. [Greek]

[30] Jackson M, Colwell J. Talking to children about death. Mortality 2001;6(3):321-5.

SECTION TWO: SCHOOL AND VIOLENCE

In: School, Adolescence and Health Issues
Editors: J. Merrick, A. Tenenbaum and H. A. Omar
ISBN: 978-1-62948-702-1

Chapter 13

BULLYING VICTIMIZATION AMONG IN-SCHOOL ADOLESCENTS

Patti Herring, PhD[1], Seter Siziya, BA (Ed), MSc, PhD[2,*], Sricharan Pasupulati, MD, MPH[3], Emmanuel Rudatsikira, MD, MPH, DrPH[4] and Adamson S Muula, MBBS, MPH, PhD[5]

[1]School of Public Health, Loma Linda University, Loma Linda, California, US
[2]School of Medicine, The Copperbelt University, Ndola, Zambia
[3]School of Community and Environmental Health, Old Dominion University, Norfolk, Virginia, US
[4]School of Health Professions, Andrews University, Berrien Springs, Michigan, US
[5]Department of Community Health, University of Malawi, Blantyre, Malawi

ABSTRACT

Bullying victimization is a major public health problem among adolescents. It is associated with poor academic performance, anxiety, depression and suicidal behaviors. There are limited reports on victimization from bullying among Botswana adolescents. The purpose of this study was to determine the correlates for bullying victimization among school-going adolescents in Botswana. The 2005 Botswana Global School-based Health Survey (GSHS) data were obtained from the World Health Organization. A weighted analysis was conducted using statistical software (SPSS version 15.0). We estimated the prevalence of bullying victimization and conducted logistic regression analysis to estimate associations between the outcome (bullying victimization) and selected explanatory variables. Out of 2,165 in-school adolescents who participated in the study, 51.3% (54.2% males and 52.2% females; p=0.086) reported having been bullied in the last 30 days. In multivariate analysis, bullying victimization was positively associated with physical fighting (OR=2.17; 95% CI [1.73, 2.73]), truancy (OR=1.84; 95% CI [1.35, 2.50]), and alcohol drinking (OR=1.41; 95% CI [1.04, 1.91]). Victimization is prevalent

* Correspondence: Professor Seter Siziya, BA (Ed), MSc, PhD, The Copperbelt University, School of Medicine, Department of Clinical Sciences, Public Health Unit, Box 71191, Ndola, Zambia. E-mail: ssiziya@gmail.com.

among in-school adolescents in Botswana. Efforts to prevent and control bullying should take into consideration the factors identified in this study.

INTRODUCTION

Where data are available, bullying victimization is prevalent globally with significant regional variations in the rates of victimization (1-2). In a study on bully victimization among in-school adolescents from five continents, Due et al. (2) reported the highest prevalence for bullying victimization among boys was in Zimbabwe (70.2%), while Zambia had the highest prevalence for girls (67%). Adverse conditions positively associated with victimization from bullying include serious injuries (3), alcohol and drug use (4), truancy (5), depression (6) and suicidal behaviors (7).

Bullying victimization is common in Botswana among school going adolescents. Fleming and Jacobsen (4) reports rates of being bullied as high as 53.0% with no sex difference (52.2% of females and 54.2% of males). They also considered factors (age, sex, symptoms of depression) associated with being bullied in their study but in their analysis they used the relative risk as a measure of the magnitude of association. Unfortunately the relative risk is not an appropriate measure of association in cross sectional studies. The purpose of this study was to re-analyze the data on correlates for bullying victimization among school-going adolescents in Botswana so that we may provide public health officers with correct results for use in interventions.

OUR STUDY

This study was based on a secondary analysis of data from the Botswana Global School-based Student Health Survey (GSHS) that was conducted in 2005. The 2005 Botswana GSHS was a school-based survey which included students in classes with the majority ages of 13-15 years. A two-stage cluster sampling design was used to produce data that was representative of students in the country. At the first stage, schools were selected with probability proportional to enrolment size. At the second stage, classes were randomly selected and all students in selected classes were eligible to participate. There was no replacement of students who were not available despite being in the selected schools. Students self-completed the questionnaires and the responses to questions were indicated on a computer scannable answer sheet.

In order to assess history of victimization from bullying, the question that was asked was: During the past 30 days, on how many days were you bullied? Possible responses included 0 days or any number of days. In terms of involvement in a physical fight, students were asked the question: During the past 12 months, how many times were you in a physical fight? Options included 0 times, one up to 12 or more times.

These data were obtained from the World Health Organization. The study was approved by the Botswana Ministry of Health. Parents were informed of the study through a letter, and students gave verbal consent to participate in the survey. To preserve individual confidentiality, the questionnaire was anonymously self-reported by the students.

Cases with missing values were not considered in the analysis. A weighting factor was used in the analysis to account for differences in the probability of selecting a school and classroom, and to account for differences in non response rates for various strata.

Data were first analyzed using SPSS version 11.5. Unweighted frequencies and their weighted percentages are reported. For the main outcome (bullying victimization), we recoded the responses in two categories: 0 for not having been victimized in the past 30 days, and 1 for having been victimized in the past 30 days. We conducted bivariate and multivariate logistic regression analyses in order to estimate associations between independent factors and the outcome variable. The hypotheses were "There were no significant associations between socio-demographic factors and bullying victimization". We report prevalence of bullying victimization as well as the unadjusted odds ratios (OR) and adjusted odds ratios (AOR) together with their 95% confidence intervals (CI).

Table 1. Socio-demographic characteristics and bullying victimization of the study population

Factor	Male n (%)	Female n (%)	Total (%)
Age (years)			
< 14	78 (8.0)	131 (11.0)	209 (9.7)
14	190 (19.5)	302 (25.3)	492 (22.7)
15	319 (32.8)	372 (31.2)	6 (1.9)
16 +	385 (39.6)	388 (32.5)	773 (35.7)
Physical fight			
No	458 (47.1)	691 (58.3)	1149 (53.3)
Yes	514 (52.9)	494 (41.7)	1008 (46.7)
Parental supervision			
No	326 (34.5)	348 (30)	674 (32)
Yes	618 (65.5)	811 (70)	1429 (68)
Depression			
No	569 (59.6)	651 (55.7)	1220 (57.5)
Yes	385 (40.4)	518 (44.3)	903 (42.5)
Cigarette smoking			
No	817 (89)	1083 (95.2)	1900 (92.4)
Yes	101 (11)	55 (4.8)	156 (7.6)
Alcohol drinking			
No	596 (75.9)	795 (78.8)	1391 (77.5)
Yes	189 (24.1)	214 (21.2)	403 (22.5)
Drug use			
No	840 (86.3)	1138 (95.4)	1978 (91.3)
Yes	133 (13.7)	55 (4.6)	188 (8.7)
Truancy			
No	665 (70.2)	950 (80.3)	1615 (75.8)
Yes	282 (29.8)	233 (19.7)	515 (24.2)
Bullied			
No	377 (45.8)	481 (47.8)	858 (46.9)
Yes	446 (54.2)	525 (52.2)	971 (53.1)

FINDINGS

A total of 2,165 students participated in the 2005 Botswana GSHS; and 1829 had information on whether they were bullied or not. Overall, 42.4% were depressed; 22.5% consumed alcohol; and 8.7% had used illicit drugs. More than 1 in five (22.5%) participants reported having missed classes without permission. Altogether, 53.1% (54.2% of male and 52.2% of female) participants reported having been bullied in the previous 30 days to the survey. Further description of the sample by gender is shown in Table 1.

Table 2 reports associations between being bullied and selected factors. Being bullied was positively associated with having engaged in physical fighting (OR=2.17; 95% CI [1.73, 2.73]), self reported feelings of depression (OR=1.40; 95% CI [1.16, 1.77]); truancy (OR=1.84; 95% CI [1.35, 2.50]); and alcohol drinking (OR=1.41; 95% CI [1.04, 1.91]).

DISCUSSION

In a study of bullying victimization among in-school adolescents in Botswana, we found that 53.1% of the respondents were bullied in the last month. This prevalence is higher than the average (32%) for 66 countries and territories from five continents (2). In Africa, that prevalence is lower than 62.8% reported in Zambia (9), but higher than 40.1% in Ghana (8) and 39.6% in neighboring Swaziland (5).

We found that bullying victimization was positively associated with reported depression, having engaged in physical fighting, truancy, and alcohol drinking. In a study of the association between bullying and psychological health among senior high school students in Ghana, Owuso et al. found that bullying victimization was positively associated with depression, suicide ideation, and loneliness (8). The association between bullying victimization and physical fighting was reported previously in other settings such as Zambia (9), Philippines (10) and China (11). In a study of the association between physical bullying victimization and physical fighting among Filipino school going adolescents, Rudatsikira et al. reported a dose-response relationship between the two (10). Previous studies have reported the relationship between bullying victimization and alcohol use and other substances (12, 13).

In this study, there was no significant gender difference in bullying victimization. Some studies have reported similar findings (8, 10) while others have reported that males were more likely to be bullied than females (9, 11). What is consistent in the literature is the gender difference in the types of bullying victimization; males are more at risk for physical victimization while females are more at risk of relational or emotional victimization (14-15).

The present study has several limitations and strengths. Data were collected through self-reports. To the extent that study participants mis-reported, intentionally or not, our findings may be biased. The study design was cross sectional which limits us from ascribing causation between the outcome and explanatory variables. It is also important to note that different studies have defined bullying differently. For instance, Sourander et al. (16) defined bullying as "an aggressive act embodying an imbalance of power in which the victims cannot defend themselves accompanied by an element of repetition." Our study only asked whether students had been bullied. However, the sample size was large thus improving precision of the effect measure estimates. That this study is a secondary analysis of existing data can be both a strength and a weakness. A strength in that the subjects' responses could be accurate as study participants may not have anticipated any links between outcome variable and explanatory variables, hence truthful reporting; and a weakness in that there are likely to be several unmeasured confounders that a primary study could have planned to measure.

Table 2. Factors associated with being bullied

Factor	Bullied n (%)	OR[1] (95% CI[3])	AOR[2] (95% CI)
Age (years)			
< 14	89 (9.2)	0.95 (0.67-1.35)	1.12 (0.76-1.67)
14	216 (22.3)	0.83 (0.59-1.16)	1.06 (0.79-1.43)
15	309 (31.9)	0.82 (0.59-1.14)	0.97 (0.74-1.28)
16+	355 (36.6)	1	1
Sex			
Male	446 (45.5)	1.08 (0.90-1.30)	0.92 (0.73-1.16)
Female	525 (54.5)	1	1
Physical fight			
No	409 (42.3)	1	1
Yes	557 (57.7)	2.89 (2.38-3.50)	2.17 (1.73-2.73)
Depression			
No	495 (52.2)	1	1
Yes	454 (47.8)	1.74 (1.44 - 2.10)	1.40 (1.16-1.77)
Cigarette smoking			
No	807 (88.8)	1	1
Yes	102 (11.2)	3.54 (2.31 - 5.40)	1.36 (0.77-2.40)
Drug use			
No	853 (88.1)	1	1
Yes	115 (11.9)	3.01 (2.06 - 4.42)	1.26 (0.7-2.26)
Truancy			
No	666 (69.1)	1	1
Yes	287 (30.1)	2.63 (2.10 - 3.33)	1.84 (1.35-2.5)
Parental supervision			
No	314 (33.1)	1	1
Yes	634 (66.9)	0.87 (0.70 - 1.10)	0.80 (0.85-1.37)
Alcohol drinking			
No	538 (69.7)	1	1
Yes	238 (30.7)	2.44 (1.90-3.13)	1.41 (1.04-1.91)

[1]OR Unadjusted odds ratio.
[2]AOR Adjusted odds ratio.
[3]CI confidence interval.

CONCLUSION

In this study, we found that bullying victimization was prevalent among school-going adolescents in Botswana. Efforts to prevent and control bullying should take into consideration the factors identified in this study.

ACKNOWLEDGEMENTS

We thank the World Health Organization for availing the data for further analysis and the students for their participation in the survey.

REFERENCES

[1] Craig W, Harel-Fisch Y, Fogel-Grinvald H, Dostaler S, Hetland J, Simons-Morton B, et al. A cross-national profile of bullying and victimization among adolescents in 40 countries. Int J Public Health 2009;54(Suppl 2):216-24.

[2] Due P, Holstein BE, Soc MS. Bullying victimization among 13 to 15-year old school children: results from two comparative studies in 66 countries and regions. Int J Adolesc Med Health 2008;20:209-21.

[3] Muula AS, Siziya S, Rudatsikira E. Prevalence and socio-demographic correlates of serious injuries among adolescents participating in the Djibouti 2007 Global School-based Health Survey. BMC Res Notes 2011;4:372.

[4] Fleming LC, Jacobsen KH. Bullying among middle-school students in low and middle income countries. Health Promot Int 2010;25:73-84.

[5] Siziya S, Muula AS, Rudatsikira E. Prevalence and correlates of truancy among adolescents in Swaziland: findings from the Global School-based Health Survey. Child Adolesc Psychiatr Ment Health 2007;1:15.

[6] Fleming LC, Jacobsen KH. Bullying and symptoms of depression in Chilean middle school students. J Sch Health 2009;79:130-7.

[7] Klomek AB, Sourander A, Niemela S, Kumpulainen H, Piha J, Tamminen T, et al. Childhoold bullying behavior as a risk for suicide attempts and complete suicides: a population-based birth cohort study. J Am Acad Child Adolesc Psychiatry 2009;48:254-61.

[8] Owusu A, Hart P, Oliver B, Kang M. The association between bullying and psychological health among senior high school students in Ghana, West Africa. J Sch Health 2011;81:231-8.

[9] Siziya S, Rudatsikira E, Muula AS. Victimization from bullying among school-attending adolescents in grades 7 to 10 in Zambia. J Inj Violence Res 2012;4:30-5.

[10] Rudatsikira E, Mataya RH, Siziya S, Muula AS. Association between bullying victimization and physical fighting among Filipino adolescents: results from the Global School-Based Health Survey. Indian J Pediatr 2008;75:1243-7.

[11] Hazemba A, Siziya S, Muula AS, Rudatsikira E. Prevalence and correlates of being bullied among in-school adolescents in Beijing: results from the 2003 Beijing Global School-Based Health Survey. Ann Gen Psychiatry 2008;7:6.

[12] Swahn MH, Topalli V, Strasser SM, Ashby JS, Meyers J. Pre-teen alcohol use as a risk factor for victimization and perpetration of bullying among middle and high school students in Georgia. West J Emerg Med 2011;12:305-9.

[13] Radliff KM, Wheaton JE, Robinson K, Morris J. Illuminating the relationship between bullying and substance use among middle and high school youth. Addict Behav 2012;37:569-72.

[14] Hampel P. Direct and relational bullying among children and adolescents: coping and psychological adjustment. Sch Psychol Int 2009;30:474-90.

[15] Frisen A, Jonsson A, Persson C. Adolescents's perception of bullying: who is the victim? Who is the bully? What can be done to stop bullying? Adolescence 2007;42:749-61.
[16] Sourander A, Ronning J, Brunstein-Klomek A, Gyllenberg D, Kumpulainen K, Niemelä S, Helenius H, Sillanmäki L, Ristkari T, Tamminen T, Moilanen I, Piha J, Almqvist F. Childhood bullying behavior and later psychiatric hospital and psychopharmacologic treatment: findings from the Finnish 1981 birth cohort study. Arch Gen Psychiatry 2009;66:1005-12.

In: School, Adolescence and Health Issues
Editors: J. Merrick, A. Tenenbaum and H. A. Omar
ISBN: 978-1-62948-702-1

Chapter 14

AGGRESSION AMONG HIGH SCHOOL STUDENTS

Manmeet Kaur Reen, BSC, MSC, APGDCGFC, B.ED [*]
and Deepali Sharma, PhD
Department of Human Development and Family Relations,
Government Home Science College, Panjab University, Chandigarh, India

In this chapter we carried out a comparative study on a sample of 140 school going adolescents from class IX. A standardized questionnaire was administered to determine the prevalence of aggression in adolescents of private and government schools of Chandigarh. The results were analyzed using t-test. Regarding the school type, there were no significant differences between adolescents coming from government schools and those studying in private schools. Related to the sub scales of aggression, there was no gender difference except for the Anger scale (AngS) in which female respondents showed significantly higher scores as compared to their male counterparts. The findings highlighted the need of intervention aimed at anger management. Workshops and seminars can also be organized for parents, teachers and adolescents on adolescents' aggressive behavior.

INTRODUCTION

Adolescence is viewed as a period during which biological, cognitive, emotional and social changes and development takes place. Because of reorganization in all of the developmental areas, young children face various behavioral of adjustment problems (1). It is often assumed that this is a difficult period of life, with the adolescents being at risk of high stress, since they have to cope with enormous changes. Some of these changes are in the physical and sexual behavior following puberty, some of the social and financial area, and some relate to decisions about the future. Thus, this period is certainly a period of change in which the adolescents are burdened by various pressures (2).

[*] Correspondence: Manmeet Kaur Reen, BSC, MSC, APGDCGFC, B. ED, Department of Human Development and Family Relations, Government Home Science College, Panjab University, Chandigarh, Chandigarh, India. E-mail: manmeetreen@ymail.com

It is very important that adolescents pass through this stage successful otherwise problems may occur which may further lead to the formation of various kinds of deviant behavior like aggression, drug and alcohol use. Erikson (3) further argues that adolescents typically experience diffusion, a strong sense of uncertainty and need to achieve a sense of identity. But at this phase of life they find it hard to do this and are always perturbed about who they are and what their future will be? Such unanswered questions might lead to frustration and aggressive behavior among the adolescents (4,5). Further, biological or hormonal changes in adolescents (increased level of androgen and testosterone) are also associated with behavioral problems like rebelliousness, talking back to adults, and fighting with classmates (6).

Thus, emphasizing upon the critical nature of adolescent stage ,it is apparent that adolescence and aggression cannot be separated. Many studies tracing the problems of adolescence over several decades have shown an increase in the rate of aggression among the adolescents (7).

Aggression is defined as physical or verbal behavior intended to harm. Aggression can either be directed inward by self mutilation ,or directed outwardly at another person. Aggressive behavior is often used to claim status, precedents or access to an object or territory (8). According to Eysenck (2), two kinds of aggression are identified namely, person oriented and instrumental aggression. Person oriented aggression is designed to hurt someone else were causing harm in the main goal. In contrast, instrumental aggression has its main goal in obtaining some desired reward with aggression. Another category of aggression is based on the initiator of the aggression. Proactive aggression is aggressive behavior that is initiated by the individual to achieve some desired outcomes whereas reactive aggression in an individual reaction to someone else aggression.

These distinctions clearly revealed that aggression is not simple but a complicated aspect. It is not a single idea but it is of various types such as physical or verbal aggression.

Physical aggression

As the word indicates physical aggression is any response that produces or is intended to produce physical injury or physical pain in the victim or damage to an object. It involves the acts of hitting and kicking (9). The large body mass or higher physical development among the early adolescents is also an important predictor of the growing physical aggression among them. This is particularly supported by Trembley (10) who studied the association among the testosterone, physical development, and social behavior during early adolescence. He suggests that adolescents with larger body masses are more likely to be physically aggressive or socially dominant and tend to have higher testosterone levels, when provoked; adolescents tend to show physical aggressive behavior; like they would hit the person who irritates them.

Verbal aggression

Burbank (11) reports that children are involved in violence and physical aggression until they have attained the verbal skills but when these are developed, physical aggression is replaced by verbal aggression up to some extent. Infante (12) reveals that verbal aggression is a message behavior, which harms the self esteem of a person and thus produces psychological pain. Broadly speaking, verbal aggression is any response that produces psychological or social harm to the victim, hurt feelings, and damage to one's reputation, devaluation that could result in loss of prize, a job, and so forth. Nasty remarks, name calling are the active and verbal forms of verbal aggression whereas stony silence or sulking form a part of passive and non verbal aggression. In general terms verbal aggression is confined to yelling and screaming at others. Verbal aggression is a softer part than the physical aggression and is generally done for betterment. As Burbank (11) reports that verbal aggression is used for escape from demanding or difficult situations, and relief from stress. In the highly competitive world of today adolescents feel a threat to their identity, so in this process of getting the attention they always try to make others agree with their viewpoints. But when others disagree, they get into conflicts, indulge in heated arguments, and show verbal aggression.

Anger

Goodenough and Gesell (13, 14) report that infants and young children respond in anger in a direct and primitive manner, but as they develop the responses become less violent and more symbolic. In early school years anger reactions become more directed toward a single person and take the form of attempts to hurt the feeling rather than to injure the body of the offender. In middle school years, the anger is shown more on verbal plane. Anger reaction is displaced on others rather than on the person himself. The study also suggested that children think themselves as bosses if they shout or show violent reaction towards their peers.

Indirect aggression

Indirect aggression means telling untruth behind the back, starts being somebody else's friend in revenge, abuses, argues, sulks, take revenge in play (9).

THEORETICAL ORIENTATION

The study of aggression is a perfect example of nature-nurture debate, which is of central concern in many psychological arguments. The question being asked is whether aggression, as a characteristic of human being, is biologically determined or product of learning and environmental influences.

At this stage the aggression is shown mainly due to the situation or environmental conditions. So, frustration aggression theory and negative affect theory explains the behavior of the individual during early adolescent periods.

- *Frustration Aggression theory*
  Frustration always causes aggression and aggression is always the result of frustration. Aggression is therefore, triggered by frustrating situations and events.

Therefore, people are driven to aggression in order to reduce frustration and thus to maintain a balanced internal state (15). Berkowitz (16) modified this original hypothesis to suggest that frustration actually produces a state of readiness for aggression, but that causes in the situation are also important. The key concept to grasp this theory is that an external stimulus leads to behavioral response. In this particular topic frustration is the stimulus which leads to an aggressive response.

- *Negative affect theory*
  It states that negative feelings and experiments are the main cause of anger and angry aggression. Sources of anger include: - pain, frustration, loud noises, foul odors, crowding, sadness and depression (16).
  The likelihood that an angry person will act aggressively depends on his or her interpretation of the motives of the people involved. It is most applicable to adolescents and adults, who think well and already know lots about the world.

Various other important theories that explain the aggression are:

- *Psychoanalytical Theory*
  Freud theorized that human are born with an instinct towards life (which he called Eros) and an instinct towards death (called Thanatos). The death instinct, Freud argued needs to be released through aggression. Freud also stated that there is a conflict between Eros and Thanatos, some of the negative energy of the Thanatos is directed towards others, to prevent the self destruction of the individual. Thus, Freud claimed that the displacement of negative energy of the Thanatos onto others is the basis of aggression (17).
- *Evolutionary theory or Ethnological and Socio-biological views*
  It states that humans are born with fighting instinct and aggression is built into our nature. Lorenz looked at instinctual aggressiveness as a product of evolution. In essence, he combined Freud's theory of aggression with Charles Darwin's natural selection theory (18).
- *Social Learning Theory*
  The theory is interested in observational learning and modeling. In this theory, aggression is initially learned from social behavior and it is maintained by operant conditioning (19, 20).

RATIONALE

Adolescence is a crucial stage that involves going through varied physical and emotional changes. One of the most important behavior aspects during adolescence is aggression which is likely to be influenced by gender, and school type. Limited work is available in this area thus suggesting the crucial need to understand the influence of these independent variables on the aggressive behavior of the adolescents.

Are boys more physically aggressive than girls? Are girls more verbally aggressive? How does school environment effect aggressive behavior? Based on study it will hopefully be possible to identify the areas of intervention further promotes the well being of the adolescent.

The following were the objectives of the study:

- To assess the prevalence and level of aggression among high school students.
- To examine gender differences among the respondents related to aggression.

OUR STUDY

The present research was planned as a comparative study on aggression carried out on a sample of 140 school going adolescents (70 Government and 70 from Private schools in Chandigarh. For the present study, aggression was the independent variable and gender and type of school were the dependent variables.

This study was conducted in Chandigarh and purposive sampling was done when it came to selection of the school and participants. In total four schools were selected which represented the government and private schools. Care was taken that these four schools represented the four geographical zones of Chandigarh. Within the government and private schools, the respondents were randomly selected. The sample was further segregated into the sub-category of gender i.e., boys and girls.

Assessment Measures

- Background information

A personal information sheet was prepared to collect the background information of the adolescents (Appendix A). It contained questions related to demographic factors such as age, school, gender, class, family type and birth order.

- The Aggression Questionnaire (2000)

A standardized questionnaire was administered to determine the prevalence of aggression in adolescents (Appendix A). The questionnaire had 34 items with the following areas: (i) general information (for example: name, age, gender, type of family, etc.); (ii) physical aggression (for example: I have threatened people I know, I get into fights more than most people); (iii) Verbal aggression (for example: my friends say that I argue a lot, I cannot help getting into arguments when people disagree with me); (iv) Anger (for example: some of my friends think I am short tempered, I have trouble controlling my temper); (v) Hostility (for example: I know that friends talk about me behind my back, I wonder what people want when they are nice to me); (vi) Indirect aggression (for example: I have been angry enough to bang a door when leaving someone behind in the room, I sometimes spread gossip about people I do not like).

The application of the test was discussed among the investigative team and accordingly changes were made. Certain statements or words in the tool that were not applicable in the Indian context were reworded.

The calculation of the level of aggression was done by converting raw scores into T scores by applying the formula given below:

T= 50+10(X-Y)/Z

Where,

X=Raw scores of the students

Y=Average score of the whole cohort

Z=Standard deviation

The previous reports of reliability (coefficient alpha) suggest good to moderate reliability: Physical Aggression (r = .88), Verbal Aggression (r = .76), Anger (r = .78), Hostility (r = .82), Indirect Aggression (r = .71), and the Total scale (r = .94) (Buss & Warren, 2000).

Procedure

The students were contacted by taking an appointment from the school authorities and permission letters were granted by the Principal to conduct the tests. During the meeting with the Principals, the purpose of the study was also explained to them.

Class visits were made to meet the students and build rapport with them. The significance of the study was also explained. Their consent was taken and background information was collected from the students. Questionnaires were administered on both boys and girls and the doubts were clarified. The instructions about the questionnaire were given to students that for each statement they have to select the most preferred option amongst the given options.

Coding

The coding format was established and worked out by the team of investigators. The data was organized through coding. The purpose was to make it easier to tabulate the information and analyze the data for quantitative analysis. The coded data was entered using SPSS 16.0 version, which is standard statistical software, used for the purpose of analysis in the field of social sciences.

Plan of analysis

The data was analyzed by computing frequencies and percentages with the help of SPSS software to compare the responses of girls and boys from different government and private school. For analyzing the significant differences in the mean scores, t-test was employed.

FINDINGS

The study was conducted on boys and girls of different schools of Chandigarh. It aimed at studying aggression among adolescent: to know the prevalence and level of aggression in terms of gender. *Demographic characteristics:* There was a total sample of 140 students. Amongst them 77 were males and 63 were females. Most of the students constituting the sample were in the age group of 14 years. Most of them were from the nuclear family and the birth order was 1st or 2nd in majority of the sample. The study had following objectives: 1. To assess the prevalence and level of aggression among high school students. 2. To examine gender differences among the respondents related to aggression. Adolescents displayed average scores on aggression. There was no significant difference between the mean scores of the males and the females, on the overall aggression scores (see Table 1). Related to the sub scales of anger there were no gender differences noted on any of the sub scales except for the Anger scale (AngS) which had items like; "I get angry easily, but get over my anger quickly.", "At times I feel like a bomb ready to explode." etc. Female respondents showed significantly higher scores as compared to the males (see Table 2 and Figure 1).

Table 1. Mean aggression scores

Gender	N	Mean	Standard deviation	t score
Female	63	49.52	9.65	.05
Male	77	49.62	10.05	

Table 2. Mean aggression according to different sub scales

Sub Scale	Gender	N	Mean	Standard deviation	t score
Physical Aggression	Female	63	15.74	5.79	
	Male	77	16.83	6.18	1.06
Verbal Aggression	Female	63	13.09	3.82	
	Male	77	13.33	3.77	.37
Anger Scale	Female	63	19.50	4.70	
	Male	77	17.64	5.28	2.17
IRP	Female	63	17.57	5.65	
	Male	77	18.12	6.22	.55
Hostile reaction	Female	63	19.19	5.57	
	Male	77	18.67	5.52	.54
Indirect Anger	Female	63	15.17	4.47	
	Male	77	14.90	4.61	.34

*p< .05

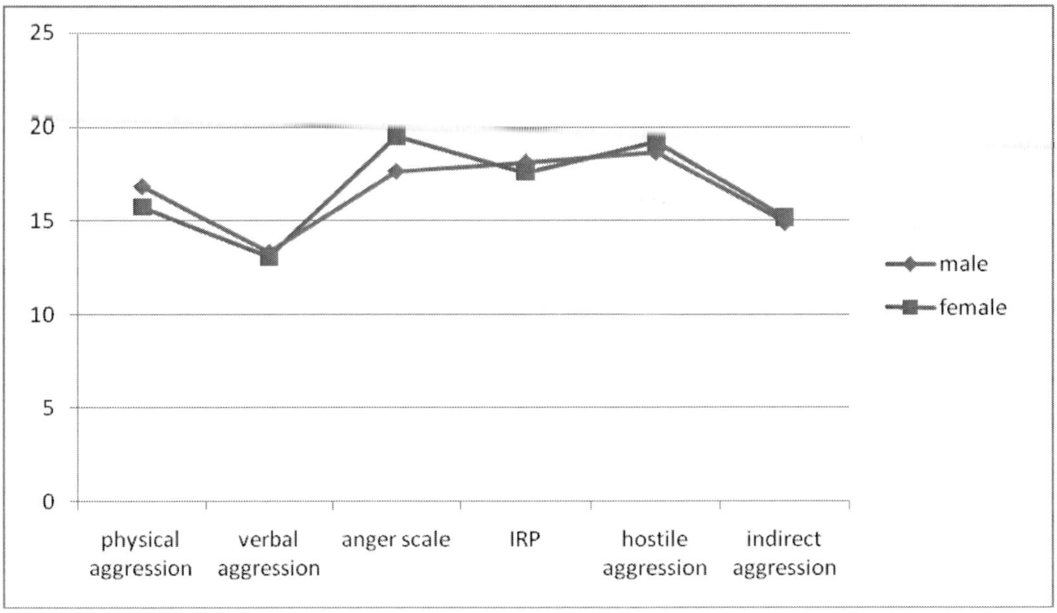

Figure 1. Mean aggression according to different sub scales of male and female respondents.

DISCUSSION

The purpose of the study was to assess the prevalence and level of aggression among Chandigarh high school students and to examine gender differences among the respondents related to aggression. The data was gathered using the standardized questionnaire. The average score on aggression and no significant difference between the mean scores of the males and the females are evident from the results of the present study. There were no gender differences found on any of the sub scales except the Anger Scale (AngS) for which many reasons can be attributed, which are as follows:

- *Changing role of society*
  Garg (21)attributes significantly higher score of the female respondents' to change in the pattern of Indian society in which appropriate sex role for females are being and replaced by more gender balanced behavior. Research has determined the anger is an important correlate of student aggression, and that there is a clear link between high levels of anger and problem behavior in school, poor academic performance, peer rejection, and psychosomatic complaints (22). Moreover, uncontrolled anger is cited as one of the factors linked to serious violence.
- *Early Maturation*
  The age of beginning of pubertal changes is gradually coming down and due to which adolescents go through varied physical and emotional changes. One of the most important behavior aspect during adolescence is aggression. As adolescence is a high stressful age, because of this adolescents become frustrated and thus show aggression (2).

- *Exposure to Mass Media*
  One of the reasons for no significant difference in the level of aggression in males and females could be exposure to mass media. Huesmann & Eron found increasing rates of aggression for both boys and girls who are exposed to media (23). A high percentage of females prefer to watch family drama in comparison, to males, who prefer to watch action based programmes.
- *Maternal Employment*
  Maternal Employment could also be one of the reasons as there is lack of supervision and parent –child interaction due to maternal employment, the child might indulge in experimentation, risky behavior and delinquent acts (21).
- *Consumption of Junk Food*
  Due to the change in life style pattern and westernization the children are consuming more of junk food, which are high in carbohydrates. This results in high body mass index that leads to attainment of puberty at an early age due to which hormonal changes take place, which may lead to aggression (24).

These findings can be useful for providing information to the school teachers about the average level of aggression among adolescents. Necessary interventions can be provided on the basis of this research. Physical aggression (as well as property violation) uniquely contributes to each of the health risk behaviors from preschool onwards .This suggests that preventive interventions aimed at physical aggression could be initiated in early childhood in an effort to reduce the risk of each of these outcomes (25).The psychologist and educators should be aware of the peer group interactions that reinforce aggressive behaviors. The intervention programmes should extend beyond aggressive children to address the attitude and norms of the peer group that may support aggression and antisocial behaviors (26).

The intervention measures that include parents, peers and individual adolescents may help decrease the aggressive and conduct problems (27). Some workshops can also be organized for parents, teachers and adolescents on anger management. Follow up activities focused on learning and practicing accepting alternatives to aggression. Focus may need to be placed on child's ability to maintain productive relationships with authority. It may also include opportunities to learn and practice constructive alternatives to non productive arguments and verbal assaults (28, 29).

The participants were only school going adolescents and therefore, it cannot be applicable to the same age children who do not go to school.

ACKNOWLEDGEMENTS

For the successful completion of this paper, I express my deep gratification to Dr. Deepali Sharma, Assistant Professor, Department of Human Development and Family Relations, Government Home Science College, sector 10, Chandigarh, under whose guidance the present work was carried out. I am grateful for her whole hearted help, keen interest, constructive criticism and valuable suggestions. A special thanks to Dr. Suman Verma, Head of Department of Human Development and Family Relations, Government Home Science College, sector 10, Chandigarh, for her guidance and help. I thank the following people whose assistance made this study possible Vandana Vohra, Rashi, Tarneet, Harleen, Renu , Vandana, Kanika, Rishya, Sukhwinder, Kamaldeep, Sofina , Navdeep and Nriti. A word of thanks to all the principals of respective schools, for giving their kind permission to proceed with my research study. I will be failing in my duty if I do not pay my regards to all our respondents for giving me their precious time and cooperation.

REFERENCES

[1] Suman EJ, Dorn LD, Schiefelblin VL. Puberty, sexuality, and health. In: Lerner RM, Brooks MAE, eds. Handbook of psychology: Developmental psychology. New York: Wiley, 2003:295-324.

[2] Eysenck, Michael W, Keane, Mark T. Cognitive psychology: A student's handbook, 4th ed. New York: Psychology Press, 2000.

[3] Erickson E. School literacy, reasoning, and civility: An anthropologist's perspective. Rev Educ Res 1984;54(4):525-46.

[4] Miller NE, Dollard J. Social learning and imitation. New Haven: Yale University Press, 1941.

[5] Glanz K, Rimer BK, Lewis FM. Health behavior and health education. Theory, research and practice. San Fransisco: Wiley, 2002.

[6] Hendry LB, Patrick H. Adolescents and television. J Youth Adolesc 1972;6(4):325-36.

[7] Zanden J. Human development, 7th ed. Boston: McGraw-Hill Higher Education, 2000.

[8] Muuss A. A concept analysis of relational aggression. J Psychiatr Ment Health Nurs 1995;14(5):510-5.

[9] Davis JQ. Anger, aggression, and adolescents. New York: Pantheon Books, 2004.

[10] Underwood MK. Social aggression among girls. New York: Guilford, 2003.

[11] Tremblay R. Testosterone, physical aggression, dominance, and physical development in early adolescence. Int J Behav Dev 1998;22(4):753-77.

[12] Burbank VK. Cross-cultural perspectives on aggression in women and girls: An introduction. Sex Roles 1994;30:169-76.

[13] Infante DA. Teaching students to understand and control verbal aggression. Commun Educ 1995;44:51-63.

[14] 13. Goodenough FL. Anger in young children. Minnesota: Minnesota Press, 1931.

[15] Gesell A. Youth the years from ten to sixteen. New York: HarperCollins, 1956.

[16] Dollard J. Frustration and aggression. Yale: Yale University Press, 1939.

[17] Berkowitz L. Aggression: Its causes, consequences, and control. New York: McGraw-Hill, 1993.

[18] Freud S. The ego and the mechanisms of defense. London: Hogarth Press, 1937.

[19] Lorenz K. On aggression. London: Methuen, 1996.

[20] Bandura A. Imitation of film-mediated aggressive models. J Abnorm Soc Psychol 1963;66: 3-11.

[21] Bandura A. Transmission of aggression. J Abnorm Soc Psychol 1961;63:575-82.

[22] Garg R. A comparative study of aggression among adolescents with respect to gender and maternal employment. Dissertation. Panjab: Panjab University Dept Hum Dev Fam Relat, 2002.

[23] Smith DC, Furlong MJ. Correlates of anger, hostility, and aggression in children and adolescents. In: Furlong MJ, Smith DC, eds. Anger, hostility, and aggression: Assessment, prevention, and intervention strategies for youth. New York: Wiley, 1994:15-38.

[24] Huesmann LR, Eron LD, eds. Television and the aggression child: A cross national comparion. Hillsdale,NJ: Erlbaum,1986.

[25] 24. Reen M K: Sexual behavior, Knowledge and attitude towards reproductive health issues of college going girls in Chandigarh. Dissertation. Panjab: Panjab University Dept Hum Dev Fam Relat, 2009.

[26] Timmermans M, Lier P, Koot HM. Which forms of adolescent external behaviors account for late adolescent risky sexual behavior and substance use? J Child Psychol Psychiatr 2008;49(4): 386-94.

[27] Lee E. The relationship of aggression and bullying to social preference: Differences in gender and types of aggression. Int J Behav Dev 2009;33(4):323-30.

[28] Barnow S, Lutch M, Freyberger H-J. Correlates of aggressive and delinquent conduct problems in adolescence. Behav Problems Adolesc 2005;31:24-39.
[29] Buss AH, Warren WL. The aggression questionnaire. Los Angeles, CA: Western Psychological Services, 2000.
[30] Buss A, Perry M. The aggression questionnaire. J Pers Soc Psychol 1992;63:452–9.

APPENDIX A

Dear Students,

You are being provided with a battery of self report tests that will assist you gain greater insights into yourself. The goal of these tests is not to provide you with new information about yourself, but rather to help you achieve a better understanding of the barriers that might be standing in your way of a more satisfying and effective life. We hope you enjoy this process of self discovery and find information that will help you have a more satisfying and effective life.

Best wishes

Manmeet Kaur Reen

THE AGGRESSION QUESTIONNAIRE

Name: ____Age: __________________

Gender: Male________Female_______ Class: _________ Section: ______________

School: ____

Birth order: 1st born ______________ 2nd born ____________ 3rd born ___________

Type of family: Nuclear ____________ Joint __________ Extended _____________

Please ticks mark the appropriate response.

Answer Key:1= Not at all like me; 2= A little like me; 3=Somewhat like me ; 4=Very much like me; 5 = Completely like me

S. No.	Statement	1	2	3	4	5
1.	My friends say that I argue a lot.					
2.	I let my anger show when I do not get what I want.					
3.	I wonder why sometimes I feel so unpleasant about things.					
4.	At times I feel like a bomb ready to explode.					
5.	I have threatened people I know.					
6.	If I am angry enough, I may spoil someone's work.					
7.	I get into fights more than most people.					
8.	I may hit someone if he or she upsets me.					
9.	At times I can't control the feeling to hit someone.					
10.	If somebody hits me, I hit back.					
11.	If I have to use violence to protect myself I will.					
12.	I get into fights more than the most people.					
13.	I have become so angry that I have broken things.					
14.	I can't help getting into arguments when people disagree with me .					

S. No.	Statement	1	2	3	4	5
15.	I often find myself disagreeing with people.					
16.	When people annoy me ,I may tell them what I think of them .					
17.	I tell my friends openly when I am disagree with them.					
18.	I get angry easily, but get over my anger quickly.					
19.	I am a calm person.					
20.	Some of my friends think I am a short tempered.					
21.	At times, I feel that life has been unfair towards me.					
22.	I have trouble controlling my anger.					
23.	I do not trust strangers who are too friendly.					
24.	Other people are luckier than me.					
25.	At times, I feel that life has been unfair towards me.					
26.	I wonder what people want when they are nice to me.					
27.	I sometimes feel that people are laughing at me behind my back.					
28.	I know that "friends" talk about me behind my back.					
29.	At times, I am so jealous that I cannot think of anything else.					
30.	When people are bossy, I take my time doing what they want, just to show them.					
31.	When someone really irritates me, I might give him or her silent treatment.					
32.	I like to play practical jokes.					
33.	I have been angry enough to bang a door when leaving someone behind in the room.					
34.	I sometimes spread gossip about people I do not like.					

In: School, Adolescence and Health Issues
Editors: J. Merrick, A. Tenenbaum and H. A. Omar
ISBN: 978-1-62948-702-1

Chapter 15

PREVALENCE OF MALTREATMENT OF ADOLESCENTS AMONG HIGH SCHOOL CHILDREN

Jyothi Manoj*, MPhil and Josmy Thomas, MSc
Kristu Jayanti College, Bangalore, Karnataka and St Joseph's Hospital, Dharmagiri, Kothamangalam, Kerala, India

ABSTRACT

The purpose of this chapter was to retrospectively analyze the awareness of adolescents about child rights and assess the prevalence of maltreatment. Methods: 300 students from two schools in Calicut district participated in a cross sectional study. The participants were 153 (51%) boys and 147 (49%) girls with median age of 14 years and range 3. Results: 53.67% of the children had poor awareness of child rights and maltreatment. The results provide baseline information on the prevalence and types of maltreatment children face. 47% were exposed to physical maltreatment, 47.6% has suffered emotional maltreatment, 16.7% sexual maltreatment, 29.7% neglect. There was no gender difference in exposure to the types of maltreatments (chi square $p > 0.05$) except sexual maltreatment where boys were found more vulnerable. Monthly income of the family and parents educational level had an influence on prevalence of maltreatment. Conclusion: Child maltreatment was highly prevalent among school children. We suggest that schools introduce interventions that incorporate personal safety, prevention of abuse and mental health issues for students. Government and NGOs should develop programmes and counseling to create awareness among parents and teachers to build up a healthy generation.

INTRODUCTION

Child maltreatment has both emotional, physical, economic and sexual consequences. However, in India, there has been a lack of understanding the extent, magnitude and trends of

* Correspondence: Jyothi Manoj, Assistant professor, Department of Statistics, Kristu Jayanti College, Bangalore-77, India. E-mail: jyothimanoj@kristujayanticollege.com

the problem (1). Children are not recognised as having human rights and adults play arbitrary limits on children's fundamental freedom. Teachers and parents have broad discretionary powers and can restrict children's freedom with little accountability. Most of the restrictions children face on a daily basis are not entrenched in law, but are part of school or family rules (2).

Discipline is something adults do to stop children from behaving in undesirable ways (3), But child abuse is more than bruises and broken bones. While physical abuse might be the most visible sign, other types of abuse, such as emotional abuse or child neglect, also leave deep, long lasting scars (4).

The impact that child maltreatment leaves damage a child's sense of self, ability to have healthy relationships, and ability to function at home, at work and at school. There is dearth of research on disciplining techniques adopted in schools in India. This study aims to analyze the awareness of high school children about their own rights to protect them from being abused. The study also attempts to estimate the prevalence of maltreatment.

Our Study

The study was carried out as a cross sectional survey in two high schools in the Calicut district of Kerala. The participants were recruited via a stratified random sampling technique with age as factor for stratification.

A sample of 300 children was selected. A self- report questionnaire was developed and piloted in collaboration with the adolescents, which elicited information on socioeconomic status, demographic profile, knowledge regarding rights and adolescent maltreatment and their experience of maltreatment at home and school. The participants were 150 (50%) rural, 153 (51%) were boys and median age 14 years and range 3. After obtaining permission from the institutional ethical review board, data was collected by the investigators. Statistical analysis was carried out by using SPSS version 17.

Findings

Reliability test of the tool suggested that the items in the questionnaire were relevant and ensured the randomness of the data (Chronback Alpha = 0.94). 83.3% [250] of the children had both their parents living together while 14% [42] of their parents were abroad and the child stayed with caretakers and 2.3% [8] had single parents. 75.7% [227] of the children come from a nuclear family, 15% [45] from three generation families and the remaining from joint families. 42% [126] of the families had monthly income less than 5000 rupee, 22% [66] have monthly income between 5000 – and 10,000 rupee and the rest 36% earned more than 10000 rupees monthly.

Based on the response to the set of 15 questions on awareness of child rights, children were classified to have poor awareness about child rights if less than 6 answers were right, moderate awareness if 6 -10 answers were right and the rest to have good awareness. The information was elicited in table 1.

Table 1. Awareness about maltreatment and rights based on gender

Gender	Poor	Average	Good
Male	94(31.67%)	28(9.33%)	27(9%)
Female	63(21%)	35(11.67%)	49(16.33%)
Total	161 (53.67%)	63 (21%)	76(25.33%)

Percentage of adolescents who had awareness about child rights and various types of maltreatment, by gender (n = 300)

The analysis revealed that 161 (53.67%) had poor knowledge about their rights. Boys lacked awareness (31.67%) more than girls (21%). When urban and rural children were compared, it was found that among the urban children 19.67% (59) had good awareness about child rights, while 23% [69] had poor knowledge (see table 2). 30.67% (92) of the rural children had poor awareness whereas about 5.66% of responders [17] had good awareness.

Table 2. Awareness about maltreatment and rights based on locality

Area of residence	Poor	Average	Good
Urban	69(23%)	22(7.33%)	59(19.67%)
Rural	92(30.67%)	41(13.67%)	17(5.66%)
Total	161 (53.67%)	63 (21%)	76(25.33%)

Table 3. Percentage of adolescents who experienced the four types of maltreatments, by gender (n = 300)

Types of maltreatment	Male%	Female%	Chi square	p value
Physical	49.02	44.90	4.067	0.254
Sexual	18.30	14.97	23.715	0.000*
Emotional	49.67	45.58	4.732	0.193
Neglect	29.41	29.93	4.05	0.256

Table 4. The factors influencing the four types of maltreatment

Factors affecting maltreatment	Wilk's lambda	p value
Parents marital status(Single parent or not)	0.961	0.765
Location of residence(urban or rural)	0.988	0.482
Mother's education level	0.935	0.041*
Father's education level	0.894	0.001*
Monthly income of the family	0.898	0.001*
Level of knowledge of the children regarding maltreatment	0.913	0.004*
Type of family (Nuclear, three generation or joint family)	0.946	0.035

It was observed that children of both genders were vulnerable to the four types of maltreatment and gender had an influence in the case of sexual maltreatment (see table 3). (Chi square p value = 0.00 for sexual maltreatment and for all others it was > 0.05). Boys suffering more from maltreatment, which is against the usual belief that girls are more prone to abuse (1-4).

The influence of various factors on the four types of maltreatment were analyzed by MANOVA. The result is presented in the table 4. The children's awareness, parent's education level, family's monthly income and type of family showed significant influence on the prevalence of maltreatment.

DISCUSSION

The repercussions of various types of maltreatment were critically analyzed. Less than 20% suffered from problems like sleeplessness, aggressive behavior, loneliness and difficulty in educational performance. The psychosocial problems expected to be present in the children exposed to maltreatment was comparatively less, which might be due to the potency in the family bond. However, prevalence of maltreatment was correlated significantly with aggressive behavior (R^2 = 0.036, p- 0.001) and difficulty in educational performance (R^2 =0.12, p= 0.00).

The findings in the study highlighted the need for more studies on the prevalence of all forms of child maltreatment in India. We suggest that schools must introduce interventions, which incorporate personal safety, prevention of abuse and mental health issues. Intervention programmes for parents and teachers that emphasize positive child disciplining practices are needed.

The investigation revealed that 53.67% of children (31.7% boys) had poor awareness of child rights. Comparing rural and urban children, we found a lack of proper awareness among rural children. 19.67% of urban children had a good awareness whereas 5.66% of rural children had good awareness about child rights. There were various factors influencing the prevalence of maltreatment.

The results showed that the monthly income of the family, parental educational level and the child awareness of maltreatment made a significant difference in the prevalence of the four types of maltreatment. Children of parents with higher education reported no maltreatment. Children who knew about their rights reported seldom or no exposure to maltreatment. Children from low income families and nuclear family reported more exposures to multiple mal-treatment. MANOVA results showed that the above mentioned factors provided an influential role in the prevalence of maltreatment. The significant consequences reported by the children who had suffered maltreatment were aggressive behavior, feeling lonely, sleeplessness and difficulty in academic performance.

REFERENCES

[1] Study on Child Abuse: India 2007. URL: wcd.nic.in/childabuse.pdf
[2] Derek K. Child social work policy and practice. London: Sage, 2009.
[3] Tiwari J. Child abuse and human rights. New Delhi: Isha Books, 2011.
[4] Child abuse and neglect. URL: www.helpguide.org/index

In: School, Adolescence and Health Issues
Editors: J. Merrick, A. Tenenbaum and H. A. Omar
ISBN: 978-1-62948-702-1

Chapter 16

ADOLESCENT DATING VIOLENCE

Anuja Bandyopadhyay, MBBS, Amit Deokar, MD and Hatim A Omar, MD, FAAP *

Division of Adolescent Medicine, Department of Pediatrics, Kentucky Children's Hospital, University of Kentucky, Lexington, Kentucky, US

ABSTRACT

Adolescent dating violence is a health and social problem, worldwide. The objective of this chapter was to identify the risk factors and consequences of dating violence, assess the prevention measures taken to increase awareness regarding it and provide an overview of the screening and interventional tools used to support the teens involved in dating violence. Methods: A review of the literature, published in the last 29 years, was conducted and the content was critically analyzed. Conclusions: There is an increasing trend of dating violence in a younger population. Consistent definitions, comprehensive assessment tools and focused screening are required to assess the actual prevalence of dating violence. Dating history, context of the date, peer influence, prior history of abuse, alcohol and drugs have been identified as significant risk factors for dating violence. Dating violence has acute as well as long term effects on the body and mind. Since, victims may not report it or even may not identify dating violence as a hazard, the responsibility of screening for it lies heavily on health care providers. Interventional measures should be implemented in a non-judgmental manner, giving due importance to the safety of the adolescents. Primary prevention programs are the key feature to reduce dating violence and require the co-operative participation of several components of the community including school personnel, health care providers, parents and the youth.

* Correspondence: Hatim Omar, MD, FAAP, Professor of Pediatrics and Obstetrics/Gynecology, Chief, Adolescent Medicine and Young Parent programs, J422, Kentucky Clinic, University of Kentucky, Lexington, KY 40536 United States. E-mail: haomar2@uky.edu.

INTRODUCTION

This article provides a critical overview of the concept of adolescent dating violence and risk factors associated with victimization and perpetration. It discusses the existing literature on the prevalence of dating violence and its health outcomes. It provides a summary of the techniques used to screen teen dating violence along with the different approaches towards managing the patients reporting it. It enumerates the measures that have been adopted till date to prevent adolescent dating violence and provide support for its survivors. It attempts to explore the potential avenues to create a more effective strategy for adolescent dating violence and the need for a formal policy to address teen dating violence. This review is intended to create an awareness regarding adolescent dating violence and help health care providers customize their approach towards the problem in their own clinical settings.

Defining dating violence has always been a difficult task. The term 'dating' may have different significance, when defining relationships between adolescents. Further, the term 'violence' may imply any shade of the spectrum varying between a seemingly harmless 'calling names' to the horrifying act of rape. The most popular definition, modeled around the article by Sugarman and Hotaling (1) stated that dating violence is "the perpetration or threat of an act of violence by at least one member of an unmarried couple on the other member within the context of dating or courtship (same sex or opposite sex)" (1). The Centers for Disease Control and Prevention- Intimate partner violence surveillance (2), further divided the acts of violence into four categories:

1. Physical violence: The intentional use of physical force with the potential for causing death, disability, injury, or harm
2. Sexual violence: This has again been divided into three types,
   a) Use of physical force to compel a person to engage in a sexual act against his or her will, whether or not the act is completed
   b) Attempted or completed sex act involving a person who is unable to understand the nature or condition of the act, to decline participation, or to communicate unwillingness to engage in the sexual act, e.g., because of illness, disability, or the influence of alcohol or other drugs, or because of intimidation or pressure
   c) Abusive sexual contact
3. Threat of physical or sexual violence: use words, gestures, or weapons to communicate the intent to cause death, disability, injury, or physical harm
4. Psychological and emotional violence: Although any psychological/emotional abuse can be measured by the intimate partner violence surveillance system, the expert panel recommended that it only be considered a type of violence when there has also been prior physical or sexual violence, or the prior threat of physical or sexual violence

The Intimate Partner Violence Surveillance: Uniform Definitions and Recommended Data Elements, Version 1.0 (2) by Centers for Disease Control and Prevention gives a uniform definition for each of the terms associated with dating violence.

A consistent definition is needed to monitor the incidence of intimate partner violence and examine trends over time and jurisdictions. Lack of consistent definitions has led to a wide array of prevalence rate of dating violence. For example, researchers have found rates as low as 9% (3) and, when verbal aggression is considered, as high as 65% (4). This is further challenged by the teen's varying interpretation of what is being asked of them. Gender-based differences may exist at the level of item interpretation. For instance, males may interpret "hit" as a closed-fisted behavior, whereas females may include an open-handed slap (5). Coercive behavior items usually include the element of force; however, males tend to describe force as psychological pressure, whereas females describe physical force (6). Widespread usage of consistent definitions would help in assessing the magnitude of dating violence and assist in directing efforts towards prevention and intervention.

IMPORTANCE OF DATING VIOLENCE

The period of adolescence is one of continual change and transition (7). Adolescents begin to search for relationships outside the family in an attempt to develop their autonomy and identity. Dating is a prominent activity during adolescent years. In 2000, 89% of adolescents ages 13 to 18 years reported this type of relationship (8). Barely eight years later, Liz Claiborne Survey (9) showed that more than one in three 11-12 years olds (37%) have acknowledged in being in a relationship; while nearly three in four 11-14 years olds (72%) say boyfriend/girlfriend relationships usually begin at age 14 or younger.

Wekerle and Wolfe (5) postulated that adolescent dating violence begins to emerge between the ages of 15 and 16 years. Recent studies show that dating violence has an earlier onset than predicted. Liz Claiborne Survey showed that one in five 13-14 year olds in relationships (20%) said they knew friends and peers who had been struck in anger (kicked, hit, slapped, or punched) by a boyfriend or girlfriend. Two in five 11-14 year olds in relationships (41%) knew friends who had been verbally abused-called names, put down, or insulted-via cellphone, IM, social networking sites (like MySpace and Facebook). More than a third of 11-14 year olds in relationships (36%) knew friends and peers of their age who had been pressured by a boyfriend/girlfriend to do things they didn't want to do. Yet half of all 11-14 year olds (49%) claimed that they did not know the warning signs of a bad/hurtful dating relationship. This may be interpreted as an evidence of inadequacy of the current interventions undertaken to spread awareness regarding this serious health problem. It was also pointed out a disturbing trend of increasing dating violence in a younger age group. The younger they are, the more vulnerable they will be to the consequences of dating violence.

Liz Claiborne Survey found a correlation between early sexual experience and teen dating violence. The survey reported that among all teens age 15-18, one in ten (10%) indicate they have been physically abused by an angry partner (kicked, punched, choked, slapped or hit). By contrast, an alarming one out of three 11-14 year olds who had sex by age 14 (33%) said they have endured such beatings. Teens who were exposed to dating violence were at higher risk for intimate partner violence later in adulthood (10, 11). Hence, this rising trend of dating violence at a younger age necessitates introspection.

Apart from vulnerability, another problem posed by teen dating violence is failure to recognize it. Pushing, hitting, and verbal threats may be mistaken for signs of love and caring and younger girls dating older boys may interpret these actions as a deeper commitment to the relationship that will result in long-term positive benefits (5). Adolescents involved in aggressive dating relationships supported this perception, with 25% to 35% interpreting the violence as an act of love (3, 12). One study showed that many girls thought that accepting abuse was a good way to secure the interest of a man with whom they were seeking a relationship (12). This distorted perception of dating violence is definitely alarming.

Dating violence is typically not a single event (13, 14). In studies of severe abusive behavior in intimate relationships, chronicity has been related to patterns of alternating cruel and kind behaviors, attachment insecurity, personality disorder (15), expectations that relationships might improve (thus barring exit from it) and a process of adaptation or accommodation to violence that blocks exit (12, 16). Appraisals of perceived control may place the victims at increased risk for abuse in the long run, as victims are unlikely to be able to control the violence as it escalates in both severity and frequency over time (16). Apart from its chronic pattern, teen dating violence has been considered to be a "potential mediating link between violence in the family of orientation and violence in the later family (the family of procreation)" (17). If this holds true, then, intimate relationship development during adolescence may offer an important window of opportunity to thwart the continuation of violence and abuse and to learn more adaptive, nonviolent alternatives (5).

VICTIMS

According to National Youth Risk Behavior Survey in 2007 (18), percentage of students between 9th to 12th grade who were hit, slapped or physically hurt on purpose by their boyfriend or girlfriend during the 12 months before the survey was found to be 9.9 (8.9-11.1). Tracing the prevalence from 1999, we see the trend rise from 8.8 (1999) to 9.5 (2001) to 8.9 (2003) to 9.2 (2005) and now to 9.9 (2007).

Overall, the prevalence of dating violence was higher among male (11.0%) than female (8.8%) students and higher among 9th-grade male (10.5%) and 12th-grade male (14.1%) than 9th-grade female (6.3%) and 12th-grade female (10.1%) students, respectively. Overall, the prevalence of dating violence was higher among black (14.2%) and Hispanic (11.1%) than white (8.4%) students; higher among black female (13.2%) and Hispanic female (10.1%) than white female (7.4%) students; and higher among black male (15.2%) than white male (9.3%) students. Overall, the prevalence of dating violence was higher among 11th-grade (10.6%) and 12th-grade (12.1%) than 9th-grade (8.5%) and 10th-grade (8.9%) students; higher among 11th-grade female (10.2%) and 12th-grade female (10.1%) than 9th-grade female (6.3%) students; and higher among 12th-grade male (14.1%) than 9th-grade male (10.5%) and 10th-grade male (9.1%) students.

Nationwide, 7.8% of students had ever been physically forced to have sexual intercourse when they did not want to. Overall, the prevalence of having been forced to have sexual intercourse was higher among female (11.3%) than male (4.5%) students; overall, the prevalence of having been forced to have sexual intercourse was higher among 11th-grade (8.5%) and 12th-grade (8.3%) than 9th-grade (6.6%) students.

Although the prevalence of dating violence among gay, lesbian or bisexual adolescents is similar to that of heterosexuals (19) rural status has been associated with a lower risk of dating violence and higher risk of early sexual debut for sexual-minority girls and a higher risk of dating violence and lower risk of early sexual debut for sexual-minority boys (20).

Another study (21) indicated that students in rural school districts are at greater risk for participating in dating violence than suburban and urban students, with rural female students at greatest risk.

PERPETRATORS

Interestingly, girls have a significantly higher prevalence than boys of reporting violence perpetration within dating relationships (22, 23) even when asked to exclude violence perpetrated in self-defense (23). Specifically, girls have a significantly higher prevalence of psychological aggression perpetration within dating relationships than boys do (22). Boys are significantly more likely to perpetrate injuries on their dating partners than girls are. Therefore, the severity and consequences of violence perpetration need to be considered in addition to the prevalence of involvement in violent behaviors (22). It has also been seen that girls were more likely than boys to report forced sex victimization within dating relationships, while boys were more likely than girls to report forced sex perpetration within dating relationship (22).

UNDER-REPORTING OF DATING VIOLENCE

Studies of college-aged populations suggest that a significant portion of young adult victims do not report acquaintance rape, specifically because of the relationship (24). It has been postulated that adolescent victims may be even more reluctant to report acquaintance rape due to past intimacy with the perpetrator or to date-specific behavior such as the use of alcohol or drugs (24). This suggests that the data on dating violence may suffer due to under-reporting. Another reason for inconsistencies in prevalence rate has been suggested by Betz (25) in an article by giving the example of two national surveys, YRBSS (Youth Risk Behavior Study Survey, 2005) and the National Crime Victimization Survey (NCVS) illustrating the differences in methodological approaches. YRBSS data are collected from students via survey in the school setting; the NCVS is completed using an interview format in the presence of family members (26), which may not provide the privacy required to disclose such information.

NEW APPROACH FOR ASSESSMENT OF PREVALENCE

Most of the information regarding dating violence prevalence has been found through surveys relying on self-report questionnaires. It has been suggested that assessment tools need to capture the sequential nature within which violence is embedded. The emotional consequence of the behavior should be measured not only by self-report, but also by other objective methods that measure the immediate response (e.g., distress) and the longer-term effects (5). Rather than focusing on 'unwanted' sexual behavior from a victim or perpetrator's standpoint, an assessment of the couple's sexual parameters may provide a different interpretation of dating violence. It has been suggested that it may be useful to measure acts of violence as well as violence "misses" (e.g., the number of times the partner was turned down when sexual advances were unwanted, the number of times the partner "accepted" such direct communication, etc.) (5).

Tracing the history Table 1 summarizes some of the studies done on adolescent dating violence over the past two decades.

Table 1. Prevalence of adolescent dating violence in various studies

First author (year)	Study design	Study settings	Subject particulars	Age group	Measure of violence and prevalence
Makepeace (17) (1981)	Cross-sectional; Using questionnaires	Medium-sized mid-western university	202 subjects 49% M 51% F	College students	1 in 5 students experienced physical violence 5.1% cases were reported to legal authorities
Henton (83) (1983)	Using self reported questionnaire	Oregon	644 54.5% M 45.5% F	High school students (mean age=17)	12.1% experienced premarital abuse
Roscoe (3) (1985)	Self report	High school in central Michigan	204	Juniors and seniors in high school	Remarkable similarity between high school and college students 'dating violence', suggestive of a pattern
Symons (84) (1994)	Cross-sectional study; using questionnaires	Rural North Carolina	561 77% F 23% M	Age range = 15-20 years	60% reported dating violence; many denied abusive relationships but recorded abusive events
Foshee (76) (1996)	Self administered questionnaire	Rural North Carolina county	1967 49.6% M 50.4% F	8th and 9th graders	25.4% reported as victim of non sexual violence, 8% reported as victim of sexual violence; 14% as perpetrator of nonsexual and 2% of sexual violence
Spencer (21) (2000)	Retrospective study	2 rural, 1 suburban and 2 urban schools of upstate New York	2094 497 (rural) 441 (suburban) 1156 (urban)	7th,9th and 11th graders	Rural students were more prone to dating violence (18%), female students being at increased risk
Swart (85) (2002)	Cross-sectional survey using questionnaires	Eldorado Park, South Africa	928	9th-12th graders	35.3% males and 43.5% females reported as perpetrators; 37.8%

First author (year)	Study design	Study settings	Subject particulars	Age group	Measure of violence and prevalence
					males and 41.7% females reported as victims
Ackard (86) (2003)	Cross-sectional survey	Nationally representative sample of United States	3533	9th to 12th graders	17% girls and 9% boys reported as victims; nearly 50% of victims reported staying in the relationship out of fear of physical harm
Smith P.H. (87) (2003)	Longitudinal survey	University of North Carolina	1569	18-19 year old women entering college	Women who were physically assaulted as adolescents were at greater risk for revictimization during their freshman year
Decker M.R.(88) (2005)	Cross sectional survey	Massachusetts	1641	9th to 12th female graders	51.6% girls diagnosed with STD/HIV reported dating violence
Marquart (89) (2007)	Cross sectional survey	National sample (United States)	20,274	Rural adolescents	16% adolescents reported as victims
Rivera-Rivera (40) (2007)	Cross-sectional survey	Mexico	7960 57.63% F 42.37% M	Age range= 12-21 years	Victims: 9.37% (female) and 8.57% (male) for psychological violence; 9.88% (female) and 22.71% (male) for physical violence
Wolitzky-Taylor K.B.(90) (2008)	Telephone-based interview	Nationally representative sample (United States)	3614	12-17 year olds	2.7% girls and 0.6% boys reported as victims of dating violence

RISK FACTORS

Looking at the studies identifying the risk factors for teen dating violence, considerable overlap may be seen between the factors responsible for perpetration and victimization. Although we may attempt to separately identify the risk factors at the individual, family and community level, in reality teen dating violence is a conglomeration of the factors co-existing at all levels.

Dating history: Multiple dating and sexual partners, earlier age at menarche and/or first date, history of dating violence are identified risk factors (27).

Context of the date: The context in which the date occurs may also have an impact on the probability of assault. If the male partner initiates the date, pays for the date, and drives, the possibility of sexual assault increases (28). Going to the perpetrator's house alone and increasing age discrepancy between victim and perpetrator (27) are relevant risk factors.

Abuse and prior violence history: History of sexual victimization before age 18 is a risk factor for sexual dating violence (27). Research has shown that young adult women with a history of sexual abuse may have difficulty in accurately perceiving risk in potentially harmful sexual situations, and therefore may be vulnerable to more repeated victimization (29). Childhood emotional abuse has been uniquely predictive of teen dating violence (30). Exposure to violence during childhood, both in the form of child abuse and family violence, has been linked to dating violence victimization and perpetration (31).

Alcohol, tobacco and drugs: Alcohol and drug use have been consistently associated with teen dating violence in most studies across the world (32-34). Early alcohol use has been found to be an important risk factor for dating violence victimization, independent of both peer and parental influences (35). Riding with a drinking driver has been regarded as a factor as well (36). Amongst the drugs, special mention may be made of the "date rape drugs", a term coined by the media to label a few specific drugs (i.e., Rohypnol, GHB and ketamine), because of the frequency with which they are used by men to facilitate rape (37). The use of these drugs for the purpose of inducing amnesia and rapid sedation of the victim is becoming more common (38). Interestingly, it has been seen that women's voluntary consumption of drugs prior to a sexual assault reduces perpetrator responsibility and blame and increases blame to the victim compared to other situations (39). Tobacco use has been implicated as a risk factor for perpetration, particularly in case of males (36).

Peer influence: Gang membership has been significantly associated with dating violence victimization in boys and perpetration in both genders (40). A sexually active peer group has been implicated as a risk factor for sexual dating violence (27).

Prior criminal history: Studies have found that history of prior criminal acts is associated with an increased probability of assaulting a partner. The relationship was greater when there was prior violent crime compared to property crime, when there was early onset of criminal behavior, and when the offender was female (41).

Parent education: At all ages, the lower the parent education, the greater the acceptance of dating abuse, likelihood of gender stereotyping, and exposure to family violence (42).

Community: Exposure to weapons and violent injury in the community was correlated to teen dating violence (43). Students in rural school districts are at greater risk for participating in dating violence than suburban and urban students, with rural female students at greatest risk (21).

Role of media: Media has a powerful influence on young minds. A study reported that exposure to violent music led to normalization of the use of violence (including violence against women) among listeners (44). Controlling for public financial assistance, relative to adolescents not experiencing dating violence, those who did were 1.9 times more likely to have viewed X-rated movies (45). The relationship between watching wrestling on television and being the perpetrator of dating violence was also stronger among females and remained consistent over a 6- to 7-month time period (46). Studies have assessed media use as a risk factor for dating violence (47).

Others: For males, having low self-esteem and having a friend who has been a victim of dating violence predicted chronic victimization while for females, living in a single parent household, having a friend who has been a victim of dating violence and being depressed predicted chronic victimization (34).

CONSEQUENCES

Studies examining dating violence and adolescents have focused primarily on physical and mental health outcomes for female victims. Limited research has examined health outcomes for adolescent male victims or for perpetrators (girls and boys) of dating violence (48).

Important sex differences have been observed in the risk behaviors associated with date violence, indicating that if girls have been involved in physical fighting with a dating partner as opposed to someone other than a dating partner, they are at particularly increased risk of attempting suicide, engaging in sexual and HIV risk behaviors, getting pregnant, and riding in a car with a drunk driver (49).

Physical impairment: Physical aggression decreased significantly across the age groups, but health consequences become more severe with age. A study found that broken nose, black eye, broken bone, went from 1% at 16 years to 4.5% at 20 years of age (50). Severe physical dating violence may cause profound physical injury.

Victims of sexual violence: Consequences of adolescent sexual violence has been considered separately, due to its wide spectrum of manifestations. Apart from the physical injury, women who are sexually assaulted experience a dramatic negative impact on their functioning. Up to 50% of rape victims develop post traumatic stress disorder as well as other psychological problems (51). In addition, victims tend to have more somatic complaints and chronic pains.

In 1974, Ann Burgess and Lynda Holmstrom described 'rape trauma syndrome' in context to the varied behavioral, somatic and psychological reactions occurring after forcible rape or attempted forcible rape. The period after sexual assault was divided into:

- Acute phase-Disorganization: It comprises of impact reactions (within hours) and immediate effects (within weeks). Impact reactions may manifest in expressed style (such as sobbing, restlessness or even smiling) or controlled style (calm, composed or subdued effect). Immediate effects may be seen as somatic manifestations (skeletal muscle tension, genitourinary disturbances) or emotional reactions (guilt, powerlessness, loss of trust, disbelief, shame, depression, denial).
- Reorganization phase: It comprises of short term effects up to 3-4 months (like generalized anxiety and fear, impaired social functioning, eating disorders) and intermediate effects up to 1 year (like phobia, sleep disturbance, increased dependence)
- Long term reactions: It comprises of reactions up to 4 years like anger, continued sexual dysfunction, hyper vigilance to danger

Furthermore, dating violence was associated with a number of risky attitudes, beliefs, and norms among sexually active girls (52), including being more than twice as likely to have a perceived risk of acquiring an STD, being more than twice as likely to have norms nonsupportive of a healthy relationship, and being 2½ times as likely to perceive themselves as having limited control over their sexuality (52).

Psychological impairment: Adolescent dating violence increases nonspecific risk toward behavioral and psychological impairment in youth, particularly female adolescents (53, 54). Dating violence was associated with higher levels of depression, suicidal thoughts, and poorer educational outcomes (54). Physical dating violence was associated with poorer psychosocial functioning, substance dependence and comorbid Axis I diagnoses (55). Abusive experiences during dating relationships may disrupt normal developmental processes, including the development of a stable self-concept and integrated body image during adolescence (56). This may give rise to higher rates of eating disorders and a low sense of emotional well-being (56).

LEGAL ASPECTS

Although, there are laws regarding intimate partner violence, a specific law regarding 'dating' violence does not exist. Restraining orders are a common legal alternative by which to seek protection from an abusive partner. A study revealed that most female intimate partner homicide victims did not have a restraining order when they were killed hinting that restraining orders may protect victims of intimate partner violence (57). However, in most states of United States, one can apply to get a domestic violence restraining order only if one is above 18 years; if one is under 18 years, then one must have an adult's name on the court papers and that adult must ask for the order on one's behalf. This may restrict the teen's options to seek help from the jurisdiction, if the teen does not want to involve an adult.

If a victim is identified after screening, they may turn to the health care providers for further information and advice. As health care providers, it may be pertinent to be well-informed about the state legal recourses for dating violence. According to the book on the "Impact of domestic violence in your legal practice: A Lawyer's Handbook" (58), providing information regarding protective order should be accompanied by a discussion with the teen of the repercussions of a legal action. Often a civil or criminal case may be followed by a violent retaliation by the abuser. In such cases, a non-legal action to keep the teen safe may be a better option. In such a situation, the responsibility for safe intervention lies heavily on the health care system. As health care providers, it is also important to familiarize oneself with the child abuse law of one's state. If the abuser be an adult, then it may be a case of child abuse. Sexual relationships between an adult and a minor partner may constitute child abuse or sexual assault depending on jurisdiction's treatment of 'statutory rape'.

Apart from legal measures, health care providers should be aware of the community resources which may be mobilized to assist the minor victims and perpetrators. Non-legal remedies utilizing combined support from health care providers, social workers, school teachers, school security, guardians, and counselors may be as effective as legal remedies in preventing recurrence of dating violence and providing support to the teens involved in it.

INTERVENTIONAL MEASURES

Screening: Studies reveal that spontaneous disclosure of dating violence is an infrequent occurrence (59, 60). According to Brown et al. (59) this secrecy may be because of several factors. First, adolescents may want to keep their dating/romantic lives private and feel shy or reluctant to divulge details. Secondly, as discussed before, they may not recognize the behavior as abusive, and may even view it as a demonstration of love. Finally, the term 'dating' may be outdated. Sex and intimacy may happen in a variety of relationship contexts, and the details may be missed if the interview is focused on dating.

The study by Brown et al. (59) showed that forced sex was screened more commonly even though it may be easier for the adolescents to disclose incidents of verbal or physical abuse rather than sexual abuse. The study found that hospital settings and female clinicians were more likely to screen for dating violence. The strongest predictor of screening was screening for other risk behaviors. Although it has been recommended that all female patients over age 14 years be screened regardless of symptoms, signs or suspicion of abuse (61) the actual screening rates remain low (59, 62). One study showed that that 52% of women reported that they had never been screened for sexual violence by a health care professional (51).

Regarding health care provider's failure to screen patients for dating violence a review of studies identified several barriers. Potential barriers include lack of training specific to this topic, lack of awareness of the prevalence of dating violence and lack of time. In a study (63), residents in pediatric training programs reported that they would not routinely screen for or manage appropriately their adolescent patients in violent dating relationships. Residents believed that although it is a physician's role to discuss adolescent dating violence, they felt that they were not adequately trained to do so. Another barrier is the provider's concern about patient's non-disclosure, fear of repercussions and non-compliance (62). However, contrary to this belief, a study reported that women find discussions of sexual violence by their health care providers to be helpful and nonintrusive. Educational, linguistic, and cultural factors appear to affect the likelihood that health care providers discuss sexual violence with their patients (51).

Several studies (48, 64) have tried to overcome these barriers and have suggested means to improve screening for teen dating violence. A few salient points have been mentioned in table 2.

Protocols that provide guidelines about what types of questions to ask patients regarding dating violence are available (64). A study (59) suggested the use of HITS screening tool with the questions "Has your partner ever":

- Hurt you physically?
- Insulted you or talked down to you?
- Threatened you with harm?
- Screamed at you or cursed you?

A study by Brown et al. (59) suggested inclusion of screening procedures as a part of training program for students, interns and residents to promote screening by health care providers. It said that board exams could emphasize the importance of dating violence by including relevant items. According to the study, health care professionals could be sensitized to detect dating violence by symposia and seminars at conferences.

Table 2. Measures to be taken while screening for teen dating violence

• To maximize safety and comfort it is important to interview in private, without the partner or parents
• Create an environment of trust and assure confidentiality
• Make eye contact
• Use specific phrases of questions which would create a comfortable disclosure climate Example: Asking a girl whether she has been abused by her boyfriend may elicit a "no", whereas asking the girl if she has felt threatened or scared in the company of her boyfriend may facilitate the truth
• Avoid words like "dating violence" or "abuse" or any such words that sounds demeaning or judgmental or anything technical and so, beyond the comprehensibility of people without professional health care training Example: Use simple questions like "At any time, has a partner hit, kicked or otherwise hurt, frightened, threatened or demeaned you?"
• If time permits it is better to use multiple open-ended questions to allow more opportunities for patients to disclose
• Do not put any blame or judgment on the victim; make it clear that you are someone they can look to for guidance
• Be aware of the symptoms of dating violence such as injuries in various stages of healing, pattern injuries where the imprint of an object, like a belt is present on the body, pelvic pain, insomnia, depressive symptoms.
• Injured patients should always be asked to explain how it happened and clinicians must be alert for answers that don't explain the injuries
• Express compassion Example: "I'm sorry this happened"
• Show respect Example: "You did not deserve such a treatment. This violence is not your fault. You have a right to be respected."
• Assess the patient's perception of abuse Example: "Some people think that such treatment is a way of expressing love. What do you think?"
• Screen for violence using gender neutral term, do not assume perpetrator is male

SURVIVING DATE VIOLENCE

Once dating violence has been recognized, it is important to proceed in a cautious manner, since the issue is sensitive. Several studies have outlined subsequent measures which may be adopted (48, 64, 65). A few key points have been mentioned in Table 3.

Table 3. Measures to be adopted after identifying a victim of adolescent dating violence

• Listen to the victim without expressing shock or judgment
• Determine the nature of the relationship with the perpetrator, and whether the victimization occurred in the distant/recent past or is ongoing
• Assess for exposure to multiple forms of violence (parental, guardian, sibling, community)
• Explain the victim's rights and options with regards to reporting, prosecution and treatment
• Assure dating violence will not be revealed to the parents or the perpetrator without consent. However, try to involve the victim's parents when possible and appropriate, if victim allows doing so.
• Perform a physical examination, if appropriate, including tests for sexually transmitted infections and pregnancy.
• Be familiar with emergency contraception for rape victims and with the facilities that provide rape counseling in your area so that immediate referral can be implemented
• Help the patient assess danger • Assess for risk factors associated with intimate partner homicide utilizing a valid risk assessment instrument such as the Danger Assessment (DA) (91) • Assess specifically for threats to kill, access to firearms, severity of physical and sexual violence, controlling and jealous behavior, stalking and harassing behavior, children in the home that perpetrator is not biological parent to, substance use (victim and perpetrator), perpetrator suicidal ideation/attempts
• Be familiar with your state's mandatory reporting laws (child abuse and intimate partner violence). Determine if adolescent is an emancipated minor and not legally reportable under child abuse laws
• Assess whether the victim feels entrapped. Being isolated from support other than the abuser can interfere with medical access and complicate discovery of future abuse. Assess whether it is safe to go home on that day.
• Promote planning for safety Asking questions like "What steps can you take in the future to keep yourself safe?" "Some young people choose to date with a group of friends they trust. Would that be an option?" "If someone hurt you again, where could you go in an emergency? How would you get there?"
• Make a safety plan for emergency
• Offer information about legal resources, such as restraining orders, mandatory arrest, police/911
• Assist in identifying trusted individuals (teacher, counselor, family member, friend)
• Assist in identifying appropriate community-based resources, programs that target adolescents including the following: Emergency housing and long-term housing advocacy, resident and nonresident counseling (individual and group) legal options (criminal justice relief, civil protection, peace order, child custody, and visitation orders), job training program

Table 3. (Continued)

•	Offer information on dating violence through brochures, internet resources (give safety alerts that computer use can be monitored)
•	Offer counseling
•	Assess need for referral to a medical or mental health specialist
•	Mobilize intervention measures for the perpetrator
•	Assess need for substance abuse treatment if needed
•	Offer follow-up
•	Schedule a follow-up appointment
•	Document all findings in medical records. S- Document what the victim Said, using exact words O- Document whatever you observed. Documentation using forensic techniques—body map with site and injury and date, photographs of injuries with written description of size and appearance, name of perpetrator, concise and objective statements A-Your assessment of potential dating violence P-Describe safety planning, mandatory reporting and follow-ups

Support groups have emerged as a key element in promoting health and providing support to the teens involved in dating violence. The groups provide a trusting and safe environment for members to share feelings and experiences and support the group members as well as encourage healing and introspection of the mind. School based support groups target the at-risk population and is tailored to students at schools who have experienced abuse. School-based support group programs, like the Expect Respect Program (66) have shown to expand awareness of abuse in the peer group, increase relationship skills and increase self-awareness. Safe Dates Program is another school and community based program which has a secondary preventive component. Secondary prevention activities target cognitive factors which influence the decision to take preventative measures; for instance, to seek help with leaving an abusive partner or to stop perpetrating dating violence. The program increases the awareness of the participants regarding their options while seeking help in the community (67).

PRIMARY PREVENTION

Apart from secondary and tertiary prevention efforts, in the form of support groups, there has also been considerable attempt to mobilize awareness and encourage primary prevention of dating violence.

Although most of these programs are based on curricula with 4 to 10 sessions that are delivered in a classroom setting (68-71), researchers have urged that prevention programs should also be made available in non-traditional settings such as housing complexes, community centers and clinics (72). Programs in special care systems like the Girl Talk 2 intervention in the juvenile justice system has found relative success in promoting protective behavior amongst the girls in the system (73).

A study by Cornelius et al. (74) revealed that, commonly used scare tactics designed to highlight the deleterious effects of dating violence often employed in encouraging participation in prevention programming, are ineffective in recruitment for dating violence prevention program. Instead, potential participants should be informed about the high prevalence of dating violence and about personal and relationship risk factors. The benefits of the prevention program should be emphasized as well, such as learning nonviolent communication, problem solving skills, and increases in relationship satisfaction (74). There is also some evidence that making programs as convenient as possible and minimizing concerns about the revelation of sensitive material by marketing programs as education rather than counseling, for example, may also be fruitful recruitment strategies (74).

A review of published literature reveals that only a few evaluations of the preventive programs have been conducted till date. Nearly all used design without random assignment to experimental and control group (68, 70, 71, 75) and measured attitude, knowledge and skills but not behavior (68, 70, 71). The Safe Dates Program evaluation (67, 69, 76-78) was randomized, controlled, evaluated behavior in addition to other aspects and was conducted at baseline, at 1 month and then yearly for 4 consecutive years. Another study by Wolfe and associates (79) was also randomized, controlled and it had a follow up of two years.

Safe Dates program provides an example of primary prevention of teen dating violence. It is based on the Safe Dates conceptual Model (78). The theoretical base for the model revolves around the key concepts of changing norms and improvising conflict management skills. Norms are instruments of social control and thus have a significant effect on behavior and conformity (80). Safe Dates program activities were designed to alter dating violence norms by increasing the adolescent's perception of negative consequences associated with dating violence and altering peer responses to dating violence. Activities were also designed to decrease adolescent acceptance of tradition gender-role norms which put females in a submissive position relative to males and males in position of power and authority. An evaluation of Safe Dates showed that the program was effective in preventing and reducing dating violence in adolescents as many as three years post intervention. Program effects were not moderated by gender or race but some effects were moderated by prior involvement in dating violence. Although it found that the design holds promise, the evaluation suggested modification in the content focusing on teaching conflict resolution skills and altering beliefs in the need for help (78).

A basic model for school based dating violence prevention program based on the examples of the Expect Respect Program (66) and Safe Dates Program (69) has been presented in figure 1, with emphasis on primary prevention of teen dating violence. Schools are ideally best equipped to promote primary prevention of dating violence. It requires development and implementation of simple strategies requiring participation of teachers, students as well as parents.

NEW APPROACHES

Newer studies suggesting methods to improve prevention program measures are warranted. A recent study identified that outcomes of school programs may be affected by format (classroom vs. small group), group type (single gender vs. mixed gender) as well as combination of these characteristics (81). A study had pointed out that no program targets couples, in part due to the flux of mid-adolescent partnership (5). It might be useful to explore these new channels while developing prevention programs to create a more effective means of intervention.

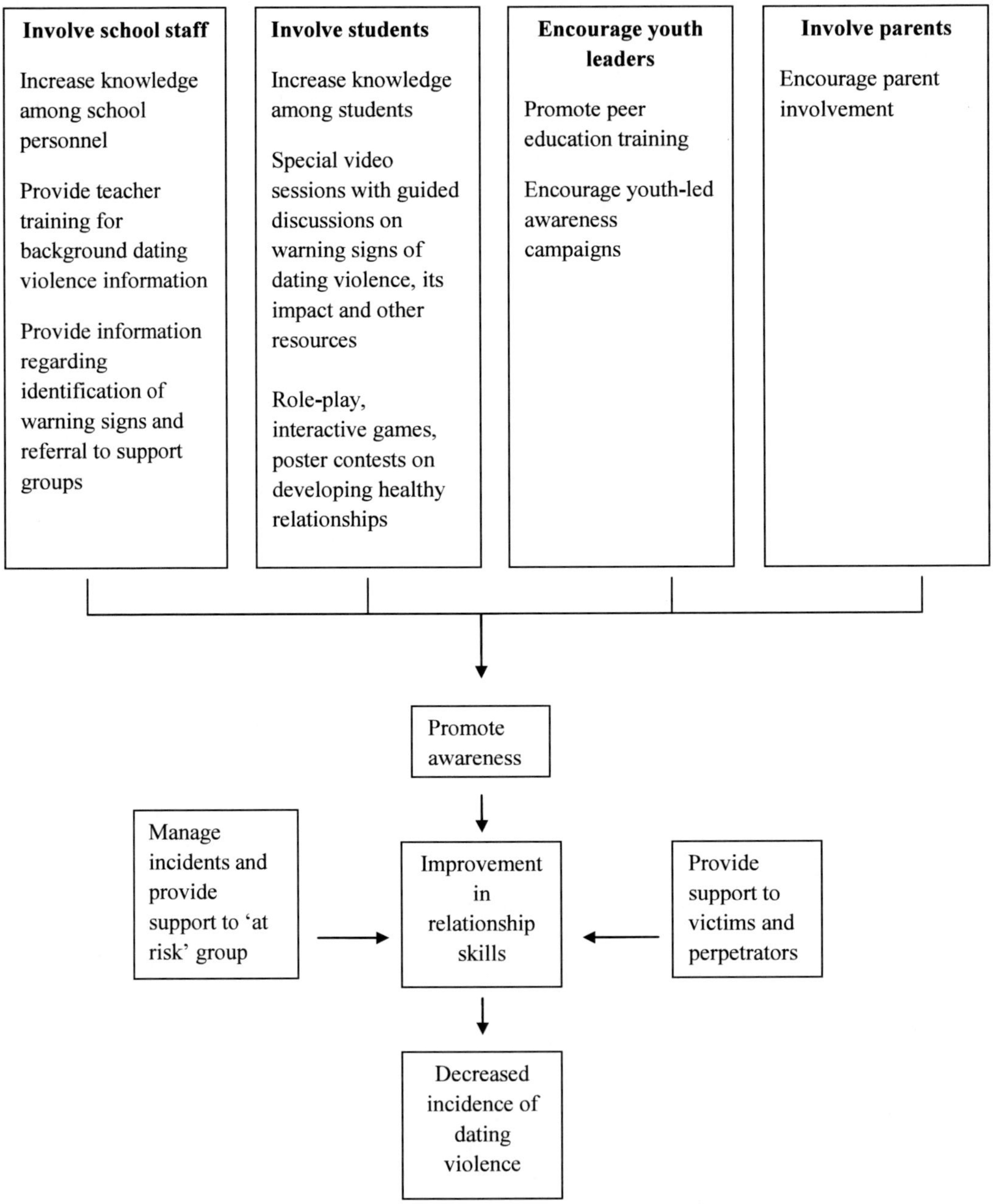

Figure 1. Basic model for school based dating violence prevention program.

Conclusion

Despite the widespread prevalence of dating violence, a study showed that 60 % of victims and 79% of perpetrators did not seek help for dating violence (60). It is consistent with the Liz Claiborne Survey (9), which showed that most children are unaware of the warning signs of dating violence. This has contributed in making teen dating violence an important social and public health problem. As health care providers, we are ideally placed to promote prevention of adolescent dating violence as well as support for the victims and perpetrators due to our regular contact with the adolescents during well-check examinations and sports physicals.

Prevention of adolescent partner violence can begin as early as age 3 or 4 years by educating patients to distinguish good touch from bad touch and to seek adult help, if they are uncomfortable with the way another child or adult is touching them. Preadolescent and early adolescent well-child examinations can include a positive discussion of how to demonstrate caring, show respect, and resolve conflicts nonviolently (64). Clinic newsletters, pamphlets, posters may help to disperse knowledge regarding healthy dating relationships.

The role of media is essential in creating an awareness of this health problem. Studies have found that adolescents use media as a potential source of health information (82). Most dating violence prevention programs make use of theatre to enact plays promoting awareness. Internet plays a major role in providing information to teens regarding warning signs of dating violence and forming support groups for the victims and perpetrators. Media has assumed this role in a responsible manner, ensuring the safety of the teens, who access this information, by deleting the traces of access on the computer, in case of possible cyber stalking.

There is a need of awareness and commitment at all levels of the society across all ages. It is the responsibility of the entire community to join hands and mobilize resources from all realms to recognize and eradicate teen dating violence and teach the young minds that love can't mean violence.

References

[1] Sugarman DB, Hotaling GT. Dating violence: A review of contextual and risk factors. In: Levy B, ed. Dating violence: Young women in danger. Seattle, WA: Seal Press, 1991:100-18.

[2] Saltzman LE. Intimate partner violence surveillance: Uniform definitions and recommended data elements: Version 1.0. Atlanta, GA: Centers Dis Control Prev, Natl Center Inj Prev Control, 2002.

[3] Roscoe B, Callahan JE. Adolescents self-report of violence in families and dating relations. Adolescence 1985;20(79):545-53.

[4] Laner MR. Courtship abuse and aggression: Contextual aspects. Sociol Spectrum 1983;3:69-83.

[5] Wekerle C, Wolfe DA. Dating violence in mid-adolescence: theory, significance, and emerging prevention initiatives. Clin Psychol Rev 1999;19(4):435-56.

[6] Muehlenhard CL, Cook SW. Men's self-reports of unwanted sexual activity. J Sex Res 1988;24:58-72.

[7] Lerner RM, Galambos NL. Adolescent development: challenges and opportunities for research, programs, and policies. Annu Rev Psychol 1998;49:413-46.

[8] Wolfe DA, Feiring C. Dating violence through the lens of adolescent romantic relationships. Child Maltreat 2000;5(4):360-3.

[9] Unlimited TR. Liz clairborne Inc. Survey on Teen Dating Abuse, 2008. URL: http://www.loveisnotabuse.com/statistics.htm.

[10] Smith PH, White JW, Holland LJ. A longitudinal perspective on dating violence among adolescent and college-age women. Am J Public Health 2003;93(7):1104-9.

[11] Taylor CA, Sorenson SB. Injunctive social norms of adults regarding teen dating violence. J Adolesc Health 2004;34(6):468-79.

[12] Johnson SB, Frattaroli S, Campbell J, Wright J, Pearson-Fields AS, Cheng TL. "I know what love means." Gender-based violence in the lives of urban adolescents. J Womens Health (Larchmt) 2005;14(2):172-9.

[13] Katz J, Kuffel SW, Coblentz A. Are there gender differences in sustaining dating violence? An examination of frequency, severity, and relationship satisfaction. J Fam Violence 2002;17(3):247-71.

[14] Marcus RF. Youth violence in everyday life. J Interpers Violence 2005;20(4):442-7.

[15] Dutton DG. The abusive personality : violence and control in intimate relationships. New York: Guilford, 2007.

[16] Pape KT, Arias I. Control, coping, and victimization in dating relationships. Violence Vict 1995;10(1):43-54.

[17] Makepeace JM. Courtship Violence among College Students. Fam Relat 1981;30(1):97-102.

[18] Eaton DK, Kann L, Kinchen S, Shanklin S, Ross J, Hawkins J, et al. Youth risk behavior surveillance--United States, 2007. MMWR Surveill Summ 2008;57(4):1-131.

[19] Freedner N, Freed LH, Yang YW, Austin SB. Dating violence among gay, lesbian, and bisexual adolescents: results from a community survey. J Adolesc Health 2002;31(6):469-74.

[20] Poon CS, Saewyc EM. Out yonder: sexual-minority adolescents in rural communities in British Columbia. Am J Public Health 2009;99(1):118-24.

[21] Spencer GA, Bryant SA. Dating violence: a comparison of rural, suburban, and urban teens. J Adolesc Health 2000;27(5):302-5.

[22] Swahn MH, Simon TR, Arias I, Bossarte RM. Measuring sex differences in violence victimization and perpetration within date and same-sex peer relationships. J Interpers Violence 2008;23(8):1120-38.

[23] Foshee VA, Linder F, MacDougall JE, Bangdiwala S. Gender differences in the longitudinal predictors of adolescent dating violence. Prev Med 2001;32(2):128-41.

[24] Rickert VI, Wiemann CM, Vaughan RD. Disclosure of date/acquaintance rape: Who reports and when. J Pediatr Adolesc Gynecol 2005;18(1):17-24.

[25] Betz C. Teen dating violence: An unrecognized health care need. J Pediatr Nurs 2007;22(6):427-9.

[26] Hickman LJ, Jaycox LH, Aronoff J. Dating violence among adolescents: prevalence, gender distribution, and prevention program effectiveness. Trauma Violence Abuse 2004;5(2):123-42.

[27] Rickert VI, Wiemann CM, Vaughan RD, White JW. Rates and risk factors for sexual violence among an ethnically diverse sample of adolescents. Arch Pediatr Adolesc Med 2004;158(12):1132-9.

[28] Megan J. Jenkins FHD. The attribution of date rape: Observer's attitudes and sexual experiences and the dating situation. J Appl Soc Psychol 1987;17(10):875-95.

[29] Terri L. Messman-Moore ALB. Risk perception, rape and sexual revictimization: A prospective study of college women. Psychol Women Quart 2006;30(2):159-72.

[30] Wekerle C, Leung E, Wall A-M, MacMillan H, Boyle M, Trocme N, et al. The contribution of childhood emotional abuse to teen dating violence among child protective services-involved youth. Child Abuse Negl 2009;33(1):45-58.

[31] Gover AR, Kaukinen C, Fox KA. The relationship between violence in the family of origin and dating violence among college students. J Interpers Violence 2008;23(12):1667-93.

[32] Easton A, Kiss E, Mowery P. Budapest Student Health Behavior Survey--Budapest, Hungary, 1999. Findings on unintentional and intentional injuries, alcohol use, and sexual activity. Cent Eur J Public Health 2004;12(2):94-101.

[33] Ramisetty-Mikler S, Goebert D, Nishimura S, Caetano R. Dating violence victimization: associated drinking and sexual risk behaviors of Asian, Native Hawaiian, and Caucasian high school students in Hawaii. J Sch Health 2006;76(8):423-9.

[34] Foshee VA, Benefield TS, Ennett ST, Bauman KE, Suchindran C. Longitudinal predictors of serious physical and sexual dating violence victimization during adolescence. Prev Med 2004;39(5):1007-16.

[35] Swahn MH, Bossarte RM, Sullivent EE, III. Age of alcohol use initiation, suicidal behavior, and peer and dating violence victimization and perpetration among high-risk, seventh-grade adolescents. Pediatrics 2008;121(2):297-305.

[36] Champion H, Foley KL, Sigmon-Smith K, Sutfin EL, DuRant RH. Contextual factors and health risk behaviors associated with date fighting among high school students. Women Health 2008;47(3):1- 22.

[37] Ian Hindmarch RB. Trends in the use of alcohol and other drugs in cases of sexual assault. Human Psychopharmacol Clin Exp 1999;14(4):225-31.

[38] Pope E, Shouldice M. Drugs and sexual Assault: A review. Trauma Violence Abuse 2001;2(1):51-5.

[39] Girard AL, Senn CY. The role of the new "date rape drugs" in attributions about date rape. J Interpers Violence 2008;23(1):3-20.

[40] Rivera-Rivera L, Allen-Leigh B, Rodriguez-Ortega G, Chavez-Ayala R, Lazcano-Ponce E. Prevalence and correlates of adolescent dating violence: baseline study of a cohort of 7,960 male and female Mexican public school students. Prev Med 2007;44(6):477-84.

[41] Straus MA, Ramirez IL. Criminal history and assault of dating partners: the role of type of prior crime, age of onset, and gender. Violence Vict 2004;19(4):413-34.

[42] Foshee VA, Karriker-Jaffe KJ, Reyes HL, Ennett ST, Suchindran C, Bauman KE, et al. What accounts for demographic differences in trajectories of adolescent dating violence? An examination of intrapersonal and contextual mediators. J Adolesc Health 2008;42(6):596-604.

[43] Malik S, Sorenson SB, Aneshensel CS. Community and dating violence among adolescents: perpetration and victimization. J Adolesc Health 1997;21(5):291-302.

[44] Johnson JD, Adams MS, Ashburn L, Reed W. Differential gender effects of exposure to rap music on African American adolescents' acceptance of teen dating violence. Sex Roles 1995;33(7):597-605.

[45] Raiford JL, Wingood GM, DiClemente RJ. Prevalence, Incidence, and predictors of dating violence: A longitudinal study of African American female adolescents. J Women's Health 2007;16(6):822-32.

[46] DuRant RH, Champion H, Wolfson M. The relationship between watching professional wrestling on television and engaging in date fighting among high school students. Pediatrics 2006;118(2):265-72.

[47] Manganello JA. Teens, dating violence, and media use: A review of the literature and conceptual model for future research. Trauma Violence Abuse 2008;9(1):3-18.

[48] Glass N, Fredland N, Campbell J, Yonas M, Sharps P, Kub J. Adolescent dating violence: prevalence, risk factors, health outcomes, and implications for clinical practice. J Obstet Gynecol Neonatal Nurs 2003;32(2):227-38.

[49] Kreiter SR, Krowchuk DP, Woods CR, Sinal SH, Lawless MR, DuRant RH. Gender differences in risk behaviors among adolescents who experience date fighting. Pediatrics 1999;104(6):1286-92.

[50] Munoz-Rivas MJ, Grana JL, O'Leary KD, Gonzalez MP. Aggression in adolescent dating relationships: prevalence, justification, and health consequences. J Adolesc Health 2007;40(4):298-304.

[51] Littleton HL, Berenson AB, Radecki Breitkopf C. An evaluation of health care providers' sexual violence screening practices. Am J Obstet Gynecol 2007;196(6):564.e1-.e7.

[52] Wingood GM, DiClemente RJ, McCree DH, Harrington K, Davies SL. Dating violence and the sexual health of black adolescent females. Pediatrics 2001;107(5):E72.

[53] Ackard DM, Eisenberg ME, Neumark-Sztainer D. Long-term impact of adolescent dating violence on the behavioral and psychological health of male and female youth. J Pediatr 2007;151(5):476-81.

[54] Banyard VL, Cross C. Consequences of teen dating violence: understanding intervening variables in ecological context. Violence Against Women 2008;14(9):998-1013.

[55] Brown A, Cosgrave E, Killackey E, Purcell R, Buckby J, Yung AR. The longitudinal association of adolescent dating violence with psychiatric disorders and functioning. J Interpers Violence 2008 Dec 19, epub ahead of print.

[56] Ackard DM, Neumark-Sztainer D. Date violence and date rape among adolescents: associations with disordered eating behaviors and psychological health. Child Abuse Negl 2002;26(5):455-73.

[57] Vittes KA, Sorenson SB. Restraining orders among victims of intimate partner homicide. Inj Prev 2008;14(3):191-5.

[58] Goelman DM, Lehrman FL, Valente RL, American Bar Association. Commission on Domestic V. The Impact of domestic violence on your legal practice: A lawyer's handbook. Washington, DC: Am Bar Assoc, Commission Domestic Violence, 1996.
[59] Brown LK, Puster KL, Vazquez EA, Hunter HL, Lescano CM. Screening practices for adolescent dating violence. J Interpers Violence 2007;22(4):456-64.
[60] Ashley OS, Foshee VA. Adolescent help-seeking for dating violence: prevalence, sociodemographic correlates, and sources of help. J Adolesc Health 2005;36(1):25-31.
[61] Saltzman LE, Green YT, Marks JS, Thacker SB. Violence against women as a public health issue: Comments from the CDC. Am J Prev Med 2000;19(4):325-9.
[62] Waalen J, Goodwin MM, Spitz AM, Petersen R, Saltzman LE. Screening for intimate partner violence by health care providers. Barriers and interventions. Am J Prev Med 2000;19(4):230-7.
[63] Forcier M, Patel R, Kahn JA. Pediatric residents' attitudes and practices regarding adolescent dating violence. Ambul Pediatr 2003;3(6):317-23.
[64] Hamberger LK, Ambuel B. Dating violence. Pediatr Clin North Am 1998;45(2):381-90.
[65] Griffin MP, Kossn MP. Clinical screening and intervention in cases of partner violence. Online J Issues Nurs 2002;7(1):3.
[66] Ball B, Kerig PK, Rosenbluth B. "Like a family but better because you can actually trust each other": the expect respect dating violence prevention program for at-risk youth. Health Promot Pract 2009;10(1 Suppl):45S-58S.
[67] Foshee VA, Bauman KE, Ennett ST, Linder GF, Benefield T, Suchindran C. Assessing the long-term effects of the Safe Dates program and a booster in preventing and reducing adolescent dating violence victimization and perpetration. Am J Public Health 2004;94(4):619-24.
[68] Avery-Leaf S, Cascardi M, O'Leary KD, Cano A. Efficacy of a dating violence prevention program on attitudes justifying aggression. J Adolesc Health 1997;21(1):11-7.
[69] Foshee VA, Bauman KE, Arriaga XB, Helms RW, Koch GG, Linder GF. An evaluation of Safe Dates, an adolescent dating violence prevention program. Am J Public Health 1998;88(1):45-50.
[70] Jaffe PG, Sudermann M, Reitzel D, Killip SM. An evaluation of a secondary school primary prevention program on violence in intimate relationships. Violence Vict 1992;7(2):129-46.
[71] Macgowan MJ. An evaluation of a dating violence prevention program for middle school students. Violence Vict 1997l;12(3):223-35.
[72] Teplin LA, McClelland GM, Abram KM, Mileusnic D. Early violent death among delinquent youth: a prospective longitudinal study. Pediatrics 2005;115(6):1586-93.
[73] Kelly PJ, Owen SV, Peralez-Dieckmann E, Martinez E. Health interventions with girls in the juvenile justice system. Womens Health Issues. 2007;17(4):227-36.
[74] Cornelius TL, Sullivan KT, Wyngarden N, Milliken JC. Participation in prevention programs for dating violence: Beliefs about relationship violence and intention to participate. J Interpers Violence 2009;24(6):1057-78.
[75] Regan ME. Implementation and evaluation of a youth violence prevention program for adolescents. J Sch Nurs 2009;25(1):27-33.
[76] Foshee VA, Linder GF, Bauman KE, Langwick SA, Arriaga XB, Heath JL, et al. The Safe Dates Project: theoretical basis, evaluation design, and selected baseline findings. Am J Prev Med 1996;12(5 Suppl):39-47.
[77] Foshee VA, Bauman KE, Greene WF, Koch GG, Linder GF, MacDougall JE. The Safe Dates program: 1-year follow-up results. Am J Public Health 2000;90(10):1619-22.
[78] Foshee VA, Bauman KE, Ennett ST, Suchindran C, Benefield T, Linder GF. Assessing the effects of the dating violence prevention program "safe dates" using random coefficient regression modeling. Prev Sci 2005;6(3):245-58.
[79] Wolfe DA, Wekerle C, Scott K, Straatman AL, Grasley C, Reitzel-Jaffe D. Dating violence prevention with at-risk youth: a controlled outcome evaluation. J Consult Clin Psychol 2003;71(2):279-91.
[80] Mizruchi EH, Perrucci R. Norm qualities and differential effects of deviant behavior: An exploratory analysis. Am Sociol Rev 1962;27(3):391-9.

[81] Clinton-Sherrod AM, Morgan-Lopez AA, Gibbs D, Hawkins SR, Hart L, Ball B, et al. Factors contributing to the effectiveness of four school-based sexual violence interventions. Health Promot Pract 2009;10(1 Suppl):19S-28S.

[82] Borzekowski DL, Rickert VV. Urban girls, internet use, and accessing health information. J Pediatr Adolesc Gynecol 2000;13(2):94-5.

[83] Henton J, Cate R, Koval J, Lloyd S, Christopher S. Romance and violence in dating relationships. J Fam Issues 1983;4(3):467-82.

[84] Symons PY, Groer MW, Kepler-Youngblood P, Slater V. Prevalence and predictors of adolescent dating violence. J Child Adolesc Psychiatr Nurs 1994;7(3):14-23.

[85] Swart L-A, Seedat M, Stevens G, Ricardo I. Violence in adolescents' romantic relationships: findings from a survey amongst school-going youth in a South African community. J Adolesc 2002;25(4):385-95.

[86] Ackard DM, Neumark-Sztainer D, Hannan P. Dating violence among a nationally representative sample of adolescent girls and boys: associations with behavioral and mental health. J Gend Specif Med 2003;6(3):39-48.

[87] Smith PH, White JW, Holland LJ. A longitudinal perspective on dating violence among adolescent and college-age women. Am J Public Health 2003;93(7):1104-9.

[88] Decker MR, Silverman JG, Raj A. Dating violence and sexually transmitted disease/HIV testing and diagnosis among adolescent females. Pediatrics 2005;116(2):e272-6.

[89] Marquart BS, Nannini DK, Edwards RW, Stanley LR, Wayman JC. Prevalence of dating violence and victimization: regional and gender differences. Adolescence 2007;42(168):645-57.

[90] Wolitzky-Taylor KB, Ruggiero KJ, Danielson CK, Resnick HS, Hanson RF, Smith DW, et al. Prevalence and correlates of dating violence in a national sample of adolescents. J Am Acad Child Adolesc Psychiatry 2008;47(7):755-62.

[91] Campbell JC, Webster DW, Glass N. The danger assessment: Validation of a lethality risk assessment instrument for intimate partner femicide. J Interpers Violence 2009;24(4):653-74.

In: School, Adolescence and Health Issues
Editors: J. Merrick, A. Tenenbaum and H. A. Omar
ISBN: 978-1-62948-702-1

Chapter 17

YOUNG OFFENDERS: PRINCIPLES OF EFFECTIVE TREATMENT

Thomas Ross*[*], *PhD and María Isabel Fontao, PhD
Forensic Psychiatry and Psychotherapy, Psychiatric Centre Reichenau, Reichenau, Germany

ABSTRACT

Correctional research has shown that young offenders have different treatment and programming needs than adult offenders. A large number of specific treatment and violence prevention programs for young offenders have been developed and applied in many countries. The majority of these programs are of the "cognitive skills type", i.e., they aim at enhancing cognitive and social skills, which are often deficient in young offenders. Modern treatment programs attend to the criminogenic needs of offenders, such as impulsivity or poor affect control, empathy deficits, low levels of socio-moral reasoning, substance use and poor problem-solving skills; a style of delivery that young offenders will find interesting and engaging; and flexibility in its administration in order to take into account potentially small custodial sentences. Programs of this type teach young offenders cognitive-behavioral skills that enable them to take their time, i.e., to stop and think before they act, in order to resolve socially complex and potentially "dangerous" situations. Focussing on treatment programs, this review provides a brief overview of the history of (young) offender treatment and some of the most common treatment and violence prevention models for young offenders.

INTRODUCTION

The Austrian psychiatrist August Aichhorn was the first seriously to concern himself with the treatment of young delinquent individuals (1). Working with delinquent youth at the city borders of Vienna about 100 years ago, he developed an influential treatment concept which

[*] Correspondence: Thomas Ross, PhD, Forensic Psychiatry and Psychotherapy, Psychiatric Centre Reichenau, Feursteinstrasse 55, D-78479 Reichenau, Germany. E-mail: thomas.ross@uni-ulm.de.

has later been described as the corrective emotional experience (2), now an indispensable terminus technicus in psychoanalytical treatment (3,4). From a theoretical point of view, he proposed a dual deficit model. He posited a failure of progression from the pleasure principle to the reality principle in conjunction with a malformation of the superego in his developmental account of the disorder. This basically accounts for lack of impulse control in delinquent individuals, as a tendency for immediate gratification persists and remains unchallenged. Excessive strictness and overindulgence were both seen as causes of the child´s or youth's failure to renounce the pleasure principle. He saw psychosocial deprivation as the primary reason for impeding the renunciation of the pleasure principle and for disrupting the internalisation of parental norms. This and the internalisation of poor parental norms in delinquent families were put forward as explanations of superego dysfunction (3). Before the "cognitive revolution" in the 1950s brought about a different theoretical view about the antecedents of delinquent and violent behavior, British, Dutch, and many German forensic psychiatric and social therapeutic facilities had worked in correspondence with the ideas laid out above. Aichhorn´s approach to treatment included a phase of getting the patient involved in the treatment process. Instead of re-enacting punishment, he would frustrate the patients´ wishes for punishment later in the process, i.e., in the case of recidivism, he tried to understand what the delinquent act actually meant for the individual, and what it stood for in the individual´s mind. Aichhorn believed that in order to renounce their narcissistic position and give up the pleasure principle in favour of the reality principle, delinquent individuals had to establish an idealizing relationship with their therapist. To establish a relationship stable enough to make positive treatment effects possible, the therapist had to be able to indulge the patient and compromise traditional views on psychoanalytic treatment techniques.

Drawing on Aichhorn´s early work, Kurt Eissler, a US-American psychoanalyst of Austrian origin, suggested that delinquents, due to their narcissistic position, are not able to establish positive transference with their therapists (5). He described the technical difficulties in treating a delinquent as a consequence of his lack of desire to change. Delinquents have no need or motive to tell the therapist what is going on in them, and their symptoms are painful not to them but to others in their environment. Furthermore, he postulated that delinquents will not be able to differentiate sources of external and internal danger, and to consciously experience and cope with anxiety stemming from these sources. Instead, in order to cope with anxiety, they tend to engage in destructive acting-out. In order to reduce anxiety, the attitude of the therapist should be characterized by qualities such as warmth, firmness, and high expectations of the person combined with clear guidance. Implicit in this is the therapist´s positive regard for the delinquent, his or her own sense of integrity and authority and belief in the possibility of change. Furthermore, he stressed the importance of capturing the imagination and curiosity of the resistant patient. Instead of applying classical psychoanalytic technique such as analysis and interpretation of thought and behavior, he stated that from time to time, real gratification should be granted. Eissler was convinced that a basic treatment of this sort is a necessary condition for aggression to translate in anxiety, and the fruitful application of psychoanalytic technique on offender patients.

Modern psychodynamic offender treatment highlights the need for establishing well structured therapeutic regimes that can support the patient´s needs to overcome resistance. This is also true for the psychodynamic treatment of young offenders. Good staff management, support and consultation are empathized; the patients need an empathetic, encouraging, and challenging therapeutic relationship and a therapeutic team that is able to convey (psychological) security. The latter is seen to be important in order to help a patient recognize and cope with his conflicts and eventually to facilitate effective prosocial conflict resolution. Recent work informed by attachment theory and its application to the treatment of offenders has generally empirically supported the notions laid out above (6, 7).

Historically, there was a second approach to offender treatment, derived from behavior therapy. In the 1960s, behavioral researchers began to aversively condition unwanted sexual fantasies, reactions, and behaviors in adults, i.e., they tried to extinguish these by means of well recognized learning mechanisms such as classical conditioning. Electric shocks or aversive olfactory stimuli were applied, for example, for the reconditioning of sexual deviant arousal. Aversion therapy was reported to be effective, at first, but scientific enthusiasm for these approaches faded quickly in the light of new findings that were more promising. Today, there is scientific consensus that, in the long run, aversive reconditioning aggravate rather than extinguish deviant sexual preferences, i.e., patients tend to get worse (8). This is not to say that general learning principles do not work in offender populations. The principle of positive reinforcement, for example, is unquestioned as an important means of enhancing prosocial behaviors in virtually all psychotherapeutic approaches to treatment, including treatments of young patients. It is important to note, however, that classical approaches to positive reinforcement such as "token economies", i.e., the simple gratification of "correct" behavioral responses, have been abandoned in recent years. This is true for both adult and young offender groups. A detailed account of the history of cognitive-behavioral approaches to the treatment of (sexual) offenders can be found in Laws and Marshall (9) and Marshall and Laws (10).

TREATMENT PROGRAMS

Beginning in the early 1970s, and in the tradition of early behavioral therapy for offenders and especially sexual offenders, scientists in Canada and the United States started to develop more complex programs aiming at the enhancement of more prosocial attitudes and skills in order to counteract antisocial behaviors. These programs replaced older ones which had mainly focussed on symptom reduction as a means of relapse prevention. In order to be effective, treatment interventions had to shift towards cognitive processes facilitating delinquent behavior and/or recidivism, i.e., denial and minimization, prosocial norm building, victim empathy, self-regulation, splitting, and the enhancement of self assertiveness. Therefore, modern offender treatment programs address a range of cognitive and social elements often found in offender populations: cognitive distortions, social skills, and low self-esteem, lack of empathy, and, especially but not exclusively in the case of sexual offenders, intimacy deficits and deviant sexuality (11, 12).

Today, numerous programs exist worldwide, and many of them are manualized, albeit not all to the same degree. By the time this paper was written, the United States alone had several repositories of model programs and systematic reviews on the Internet, e.g., published by the US National Registry of Effective Programs and Practice (SAMHSA's National Registry of Evidence-based Programs and Practices [NREPP] at http://nrepp.samhsa.gov; a model programs guide, published by the US Office of Juvenile Justice and Delinquency Prevention (OJJDP Model Program guide -Developmental Services group at http://www.ojjdp.gov/mpg/; or a web page with valuable information on blueprint programs including programs for violence prevention (Blueprints for healthy youth development at http://www.blueprintsprograms.com). Individual programs comprise different types of intervention for different offender types aiming at a range of life domains among various settings: Program types are prevention, intervention, and suppression programs; Settings can be structured along a continuum of institutionalisation: Correctional (highly institutionalised) programs; mental health programs, and non-institutionalised community programs. Offender types are grouped by age, risk (violent/non-violent), and degree of offender organisation, i.e., programs primarily devised for individuals or gang-related programs; school and after-school programs, and specialized interventions on individual, family, and peer group levels.

PRINCIPLES OF EFFECTIVE INTERVENTION

Drawing on the intensive research conducted predominantly by Andrews and colleagues since the beginning of the 1990s, a number of principles of effective correctional intervention have been formulated (13-15):

- Correctional intervention should make use of structured and validated risk-assessment. The implementation of a complete system of continuous offender risk screening and need assessments is better than the application of isolated instruments or procedures. Assessing offenders in a reliable and valid manner is regarded as a prerequisite for effective treatment, management and supervision of offenders. Furthermore, assessments should be made by staff who is well trained in the administration of tools and instruments; and there should be written accounts or protocols of the procedures that are applied.
- Clients should be assigned to treatment according to the risk principle, i.e., intensive services should be reserved for moderate and high risk cases, and never for low risk cases. Treatment targets must be strongly related to the criminogenic needs of the target group (need principle) Criminogenic needs are defined as individual dynamic factors empirically associated with risk for (re)-offending, e.g., antisocial attitudes and values, lack of problem solving skills, substance abuse, employment status, or low educational and vocational achievement.
- Cognitive behavioral interventions are the methods of choice, if they are administered in a way that matches the intellectual and emotional skills of their clients (responsivity principle).
- Managers and supervisors should attend to the relationship and structural skills of service delivery staff.
- Reinforcement of relationship and structural skills on a regular basis will help maintain primary treatment effects.
- The dosage of service delivery must be sufficiently high. For example, high risk offenders need significantly more initial structure and services than low-risk offenders. This claim is especially true for the management of day time activities, which should be occupied with delineated routine (employment, education, therapy) and other appropriated services (physical exercise, etc.).

- Treatment will work better if the management policy is supportive. Monitoring, feedback, and corrective action routine should be active ingredients of the management strategy in correctional services.
- Staff should relate to offenders in interpersonally sensitive and constructive ways to enhance intrinsic motivation because lasting behavioral change will not occur if intrinsic motivation for change is low. In recent years, motivational interviewing has been described as a technique to help clients enhance motivation for treatment. Feelings of ambivalence that usually accompany both phases of the decision process that eventually results in adherence to treatment and treatment itself, can be explored by motivational interviews. Essentially, methods of communication (e.g., Socratic questioning) are used to help clients think about why they feel that treatment is not what they want. There is reason to assume that motivational interviewing reaches its ends, i.e., helps effectively enhance motivation for initiating and maintaining self-referential processes that might eventually lead to more pro-treatment attitudes (16).
- The probability for change to occur is strongly influenced by the quality of relationship experiences an offender is making in his present environment, i.e., with probation officers, treatment providers, and institution staff. Therefore, ongoing positive reinforcement of perceived behavioral change both in correctional institutions and natural communities is regarded as a cornerstone of the maintenance and improvement of treatment effects coming from different sources, i.e., cognitive behavioral therapy, individual and/or counselling and therapy, or interpersonal skills training.

It is not far-fetched to say that there is a general rule to potential effectiveness of intervention programs. The outcome of intervention depends on the degree to which individual risk factors for violence match with the treatment components offered by the program. Treatment effects are additive. For example, programs taking into account two Andrews principles tend to have better outcomes than those focussing on one, and those who focused on three principles were better than others focussing on only two (17-19). Thus, there is a statistical relationship in the number of risk factors under treatment and the potential outcome of the program. Furthermore, the effectiveness of treatment programs depends on the quality of the program itself (evidence based treatment with well trained mental health personnel), the availability of supplemental services (e.g., individual psychotherapeutic treatment), the optimal service amount (50 or more contact hours), appropriate clients (according to risk-needs analyses). In comparison with untreated controls with average recidivism rates of 40%, Lipsey and co-workers (18, 20) expect roughly 20% recidivism for youth under the best available treatment conditions. In other words, if all relevant known factors are taken into consideration, and optimal treatment can be delivered, recidivism may be reduced by approximately 50%.

BEST PRACTICE PROGRAMS

The vast majority of treatment programs for young offenders to date is of a cognitive-behavioral type. In a meta-analysis of 509 juvenile justice programs, Lipsey (21) identified five main features of effective juvenile delinquency prevention and treatment programs:

- The primary service, i.e., the therapeutic element in it is effective, independent of its use with another intervention. In other words, the therapeutic program used must be effective for the target group.
- Supplementary services: Adding another service component to primary service often increases the effectiveness of the intervention.
- Treatment amount: The amount of service frequency must be sufficient, as indicated by service frequency, program duration, and program quality.
- Treatment quality: Service quality and the quality of implementation influence effectiveness.
- Youth risk level: Programs are generally more effective with high-risk offenders than for low-risk offenders.

Lipsey´s work also makes clear that the configurations of programs have a considerable impact on their effectiveness. Since many juvenile delinquency prevention and treatment programs are not large-scale and multi-systemic including a combination of effective individual, family, educational and vocational interventions, these programs will be less effective, even if they use single components which are typically regarded as adequate treatments for young offenders.

There are three major program effectiveness criteria: The type of program, fidelity of program implementation, and risk level. About 40% of the variation in recidivism is associated with the type of program, another 40% of the total value of a program is associated with the quality of program implementation, which is measured in terms of frequency and duration of the program (25%), and quality of service (15%). The risk level accounts for roughly 20% of the variation, i.e., programs addressing high-risk subjects are usually more effective than those addressing youth with low risk of delinquency and/or violence.

Based on his meta-analyses of programs for general delinquents, Lipsey grouped programs according to their relative effectiveness for prevention subjects, juvenile offenders on probation, and institutionalised offenders. For example, for juvenile probationers, he divided his database into three main categories, on the basis of their average effects: above-average effects, average effects, and below-average effects. Among the services with above average effects count cognitive-behavioral therapy, group counselling, vocational training, mentoring, and some forms of sex offender treatment and drug abuse treatment. Average effects are associated with family counselling or therapy, individual counselling or therapy, life skills enhancement, multi-systemic therapy, and educational intervention. Below average effects score all programs with recreation components, challenge programs, intensive supervision, and restitution. Finally, there is a number of interventions that will at best render no rehabilitative effects at all, or make things even worse. Among these count punishment regimes for juvenile offenders, scared straight programs, boot camps, large custodial facilities, long terms of confinement, curfew laws, and restrictive out of home placement for mental health treatment, psychiatric hospitalisation, and placements in residential treatment centres (22).

ADULT AND YOUTH OFFENDER PROGRAMS

While adult and young offender treatment including cognitive-behavioral treatment approaches using manualized programs have the same roots, different developmental paths have been pursued especially after Andrews published his principles of effective correctional intervention in the early 1990s (13). It has since been clear that young offenders have somewhat different treatment and programming needs than adult offenders. As both juvenile and adult offender programs draw on essentially the same knowledge base in criminology and forensic psychology, similarities prevail, especially as far as the structural makeup of best practice programs is concerned. For example, key structural components of cognitive-behavioral programs for both adults and young offenders include a shared set of criminogenic needs, such as impulsivity or poor affect control, empathy deficits, low levels of socio-moral reasoning, substance use and poor problem-solving skills. A style of delivery that participants will find interesting and engaging is not only important for young offenders, because offender groups tend to suffer from boredom, especially when they are in custody. However, owing to the ground breaking conceptual work of Andrews and co-workers (13-15), the application of meta-analysis as a method for the comparison of large samples of treatment studies (23), and the pioneering scientific work of key researchers in the field it has recently been possible to describe an array of age-related risk factors for violence and general delinquency in youth (see the paragraphs above, for relevant literature). These risk factors must be met if a program is to operate effectively. Therefore, programs aiming at the prevention and reduction of crime and violence in juveniles must be broader than those of adult offenders, using several structural elements related to the current developmental stage of the young person. In youth, parallel, where possible multi-systemic interventions on individual, vocational, peer group, community and family levels are indicated. In adult offenders, some target areas of intervention will inevitably differ from those aimed at juveniles, i.e., family (especially parents) and peer group interventions, and schooling or vocational training. Furthermore, the level of legal sanctioning is generally higher with adults than with youth, and offender careers are more visible. Adults will therefore spend more time in correctional facilities with lesser chances to participate in effective community programs.

AN EXAMPLE

The Reasoning and Rehabilitation Program (24) is a multifaceted, cognitive-behavioral program designed to teach juvenile and adult offenders cognitive skills and values that are essential for prosocial competence. The program was devised about 30 years ago and continuously updated with research findings. It is based on more than 100 studies that have yielded substantial reductions of re-offending. To date, the program has been delivered to more than forty thousand offenders world-wide. It has its roots in Canada, where about 8000 serious offenders in 47 penitentiaries have participated in the program. R&R has been applied across the spectrum of offender types: children in schools deemed at risk for offending; chronically recidivistic adult offenders; alcohol and drug-abusing offenders; violent offenders; property offenders; car thieves; child and spouse abusers; sex offenders, and white collar criminals. R&R is now being conducted in secure forensic psychiatric facilities all over the English speaking world, Germany, Spain, the Netherlands, and the Baltic States.

The program consists of nine interrelated modules: problem solving, social skills, values enhancement, critical reasoning, negotiation skills, creative thinking, the management of emotions, cognitive exercises, and skills in review. Program targets are:

- The enhancement of self-control: offenders are taught to stop and think before they act; to consider all the consequences before making decisions; to formulate (future) plans; to use thinking techniques to control their emotions and their behavior.
- Meta-cognition: Offenders are encouraged to critically assess their own thinking; to realize that how they think determines what they think, how they feel and how they behave. Thinking strategies are taught as a means of self-regulating their behavior.
- Critical reasoning: Offenders are instructed how to think logically, objectively, and rationally without distorting the facts or externalising the blame.
- Social skills: Utilizing a modification of a structured learning therapy program (25), skills are taught which will help offenders achieve positive reinforcement rather than rejection in social situations (e.g., responding to criticism or negotiating instead of demanding).
- Interpersonal cognitive problem solving skills: offenders are taught how to analyse and to understand the emotional content of interpersonal problems, how to consider other people´s values, behavior and feelings, and how to recognize how their behavior affects other people and why others respond to them as they do.
- Creative thinking: offenders often have a rather rigid thinking style (conceptual rigidity). They are thus taught alternative thinking, i.e., how to consider alternative, prosocial rather than antisocial ways of responding to the problems they experience.
- Social perspective taking: the emphasis is on other people´s views, feelings, and thoughts, i.e., the development of empathy.
- Values enhancement: group discussion techniques are used and a number of commercially available games to teach values. The aim is to move the offender from a rather egocentric world view to a consideration of the needs of others.
- Emotional management: Anger management techniques were adapted to help offenders down-regulate excessive emotional arousal. The focus is on control of negative and the build-up of positive emotions.

The content of R&R is taught in 35 group sessions of two hours duration, the frequency is between two to four sessions a week. Some sessions require preparation on behalf of the participants. The encouragement of group activities based on great variety of working materials is the core technique to promote behavioral change: role-playing, thinking games, learning exercises with and without video-feedback, and related cognitive exercises.

There is a considerable body of empirical evidence for the effectiveness of the R&R program. As an example of the most compelling evidence of its effectiveness, Tong and Farrington (26) provided a meta-analysis of sixteen evaluations in four countries, involving

26 separate comparisons in which experimental and control groups were compared. Overall, there was a 14% reduction of recidivism for program participants compared with controls. The program was effective in community and institutional settings, and for relatively low-risk and high-risk offenders.

PROGRAMS BASED ON OTHER THAN COGNITIVE-BEHAVIORAL THEORY

The vast majority of anglo-american research on psychological treatment programs of juvenile and adult offenders encompass programs devised and delivered in the cognitive-behavioral tradition. This is not surprising given the fact that cognitive-behavioral research and treatment have been stimulating an impressive bulk of data on treatment effectiveness. Research on programs with other theoretical underpinnings, including the psychodynamic group approach, has been lagging behind. There are good reasons for this, as we will demonstrate on the example of psychodynamically oriented treatment. Personal factors of potential program tutors might play a role. Psychodynamic as compared to cognitive-behavioral therapists are on average less research oriented. Issues related to the scientific integrity of the research process have been described in this context, i.e., there has been an ongoing debate about adequate operationalizations of psychodynamic concepts. Furthermore, there might be a bias toward the publication of large-scale quantitative studies which have typically been conducted by cognitive-behavioral research personnel as compared to small qualitative individual case studies which are often preferred by psychodynamic researchers and therapists. During the last 20 years, however, psychodynamically oriented research groups have developed both individual (27, 28) and group treatments for patient groups with personality disorders who are usually regarded as difficult to treat, i.e., patients with borderline and antisocial personality disorders. The group treatment with probably the highest propensity to be effective with juvenile offender samples is mentalization based treatment (MBT) (29).

TRANSFERENCE FOCUSED PSYCHOTHERAPY (TFP)(27)

TFP is a highly structured psychodynamic individual treatment based on Otto Kernberg´s object relations model of Borderline Personality Disorder (27, 30). Although originally conceptualised as an individual treatment, TFP elements have recently been adapted to a group format in forensic settings. The results are promising in that the concepts of TFP apparently help promote an understanding of individual patients as they relate to others in complex group settings (31).

In TFP, the focus is on the interaction between the patient and the therapist, and an emphasis is placed on the current moment rather than the past. Based on early relationships with caregivers and related attachment figures, the patients' unintegrated and/or split off internal representations of self and others will be activated, made conscious and reflected upon. The aim is to help the patient integrate these representations into a more complex, i.e., a more mature structure of personality. Ideally, TFP helps patients create a more coherent sense of self, to overcome splitting and to build more positive representations of self and others. The therapist´s role is to perceive and experience the patient´s representation of the interaction in the transference relationship, and to neutrally observe and command on it without normative evaluation, or judgment. TFP has been adapted for offender populations (TFFP; Transference Focused Forensic Psychotherapy) and there are a number of pilot studies suggesting positive effects for both patients and institutional staff (32).

There is a growing body of research supporting the efficacy of TFP. For example, Clarkin et al. (28) examined the efficacy of TFP in comparison with Dialectical Behavior Therapy and Dynamic Supportive Treatment. The results indicated that although all three therapeutic approaches were effective in fostering global improvement in the symptoms of borderline personality disorder, TFP was effective in more borderline characteristics examined than either of the other two approaches. There are limitations, however, to the interpretation of these results, because patients in the TFP-condition received more individual therapy than those in the other two research groups.

MENTALIZATION BASED TREATMENT (MBT) (29)

MBT is a manualized psychodynamic group and individual treatment program for patients with borderline personality disorder, developed by Fonagy and Bateman (29, 33). The core concept of this treatment is mentalization, i.e., the capacity of humans to interpret actions of oneself and others on the basis of intentional states such as beliefs, goals, purposes, reasons, feelings, or desires. Due to disorganized attachment representations, which are often found in patients with borderline personality disorder, they tend to have limited mentalization capacity. This is also thought to be true for most offender patients. The aim of treatment is to increase mentalization in order to improve affect regulation, interpersonal functioning, and the ability to pursue life goals. The therapeutic focus is on the patient´s current present state rather than the past. During sessions the therapist seeks to activate the patients´ attachment systems, and to encourage them to create and to emotionally experience safe bonds with both the therapist and the other group members. If these processes are made accessible for conscious reflection, a psychological basis for the formation of a secure attachment relationship is provided. Thus, it will be safe for the patient to explore the mind of the other, to confront negative affect, and to understand the intentional nature of interpersonal relationships.

According to mentalization theory, the improvement of mentalization capacity of offender patients will help them perceive others as intentional psychological beings who do not pose a threat to their psychological integrity. Mentalization is also thought help them reflect the destructive nature of their violence on the mind of others. Thus, MBT will eventually enhance empathy and thus impede offenders from engaging in violence as a means of interpersonal conflict resolution, or from acting out negative mental states otherwise. Fonagy and co-workers have conducted extensive outcome research on MBT for borderline personality disorder. Compared to treatment as usual, MBT is clearly superior (34). Furthermore, MBT is without doubt a promising approach to the prevention of violence and the treatment of offender groups, including juvenile offenders (35-38).

TREATMENT EFFECTS

The effectiveness of treatment for the reduction of recidivism has been shown in hundreds if not thousands of studies, and the magnitude of effects at least equals those of many other treatments in somatic medical science (39, 40). The average effect size of all approaches to offender treatment is approximately r = .10, i.e., a reduction of recidivism in treated offenders of 10% as compared to untreated offenders (8, 13, 41-46). Although this effect size is rather moderate compared to the average effect of psychotherapy with other in- and outpatient groups (approximately r = .80) (47), it is highly significant with respect to the avoidance of serious harm inflicted upon victims and societies at large. Furthermore, treatment is cost-effective. For example, Welsh and Farrington's (48) study on the cost-benefit ratio of offender treatment reported a ratio of 1 to 1.13 - 7.14 in favour of the treatment condition. Offender treatment programs that take into account the principles of risk, need, and responsivity (13) usually do better than other approaches, approximating average effect sizes of r = .30 (17,21, 49-52). Sexual offender treatment is probably even more effective than the treatment of other (violent) offenders. For example, the meta-analysis of Lösel and Schmucker (52) included 69 studies on N = 22,181 sexual offenders and reported a reduction of recidivism in sexual delinquency of roughly 40% in treated compared to untreated individuals. There is good reason to assume that treatment of offenders is most effective when they are treated as youth, regardless of the type of index crime they have committed (20, 53). Recent research on the treatment of juvenile delinquents show high average effect sizes between r = .30 (49), r = .37 (51), and r = .43 (54). Effect sizes under the best theoretically available treatment conditions approximate r = .50 (21).

LIMITATIONS

Although there can be no doubt that the cognitive-behavioral group program approach to the prevention and treatment of juvenile offenders has been effective, there are several limitations to this approach. For example, programs tend to focus on the reduction and elimination of dynamic risk factors by teaching offenders how to avoid recidivism (avoidance goals). They usually do not focus on the flipside of the same coin, namely on the positive human goals or goods all humans seek in order to live satisfying and good lives (approach goals; Ward and co-workers have conceptualised this idea in a theory emphasising goal-directed behavior and they have put forward ten primary human goods, sought by all humans and needed for psychological well-being; for details on this theory see Ward and Brown (55); Ward and Gannon (56). The inclusion of such approach goals in existing best practice programs might help open up new perspectives on improving manualized treatments for young and adult offenders.

We also know that some (early) intervention programs could not maintain initial positive effects in the long run. One reason for this was that they tended to be repetitious and boring, with too many predefined manualized elements to be complied with and too little space for spontaneous individual input. Although modern program makers have learned from these problems and have therefore introduced systematic elements to keep participants interested, some of these problems remain. Furthermore, programs are better when implemented from and monitored by researchers rather than practitioners (18, 20, 21). It is obvious, however, that for practical reasons not all programs can be accompanied by research personnel.

Rather than a critique of manualized cognitive-behavioral programs as such, we see a rather self-made limitation to the effective development of potential alternative treatment strategies for young and adult offenders. Although conceptual work in treatments of other than the cognitive-behavioral type is quite elaborate and well advanced, these approaches are still underrepresented in the modern treatment literature.

FUTURE PERSPECTIVES

In order to make offender treatment programs even more effective than they are, the following main options should be taken into account. First, research on the selective effectiveness of individual program components should be intensified. If new programs are designed, they should be tested based on intervention components that are significantly associated with effect sizes across studies. We know that not all program components are equally effective. For example, Landenberger and Lipsey (17) reported that in order to be effective, (cognitive-behavioral) programs must contain modules teaching interpersonal problem solving skills and anger control techniques, whereas unsuccessful programs employed activities aimed at getting offenders to consider the impact of their behavior on their victims (victim impact) and simple reward and penalty schemes designed to reinforce appropriate behavior (behavior modification).

Second, if adequately adapted for the needs of young offender treatment, and implemented in a supplementary and innovative way, programs might profit from the findings of general psychological science (57).

Third, prevention and treatment programming priorities should be defined with respect to current advances in the study of age-related risk factors (58-61). From these it follows that early intervention with young children should target early delinquent behaviors associated with individual risk factors (i.e., hyperactivity, impulsivity, and attention problems), drug use, aggressive behavior, family poverty, and effective parenting with antisocial parents. Interventions for adolescents should work towards loosening offender's affiliation to antisocial peers; one focus should lie on the reduction of general involvement in delinquency, another one on the avoidance of physical violence. Pro-social ties should be strengthened at this time, improvement of mental health and relationships with parents are other issues to be taken into account. From a programmatic point of view, programs for adolescents must be systemic and multi-topic, i.e., it should comprise specific interventions on the individual, family, school, peer, and, where possible, on community level (18).

Fourth, program makers should also take a look on potential protective factors for delinquency. For example, Loeber and colleagues have conceptualised factors that predict a low probability of offending among youth exposed to risk factors and they describe factors that promote desistance. In their latest analyses, they demonstrate how protective or promotive factors have main effects in essentially the same way as risk factors, i.e., the presence of protective factors can counter-balance the detrimental effects of risk factors (61). In a study about common risk and protective factors in successful prevention programs, Durlak (62) reviewed a total of 1,200 prevention studies. Among the most important protective factors for behavior problems, school failure, physical health, physical injury and abuse and adolescent pregnancy count personal and social skills and self-efficacy (individual level), general (pro-social) support, high social norms and effective social policies (community level), good parent-child relationship (family level), high quality schools (school level), and positive role-models (peer level).

Fifth, it should be borne in mind, that treatment effects accumulate with the inclusion of individual treatment, and other supplemental services are a necessary condition for maintaining long term effects of offender treatment. In addition to sound psychological in-patient treatment, an elaborated model of after-care after release from prison or from forensic psychiatry is indispensable.

Finally, effective comprehensive strategies on preventing crime and treating juvenile offenders need to be supported by scientists and further developed. Best practice programs will not be as effective as they could be if they are not embedded in a well functioning and benevolent network of care-takers on different levels of intervention. Therefore, a strong involvement of scientists and practitioners in the development and application of social prevention and treatment policies is needed.

REFERENCES

[1] Aichhorn A. Verwahrloste Jugend; Die Psychoanalyse in der Fürsorgeerziehung: 10 Vorträge zur ersten Einführung (11. ed., 2005). [Neglected Youth; Psychoanalysis in child care and education: 10 introductory papers] Bern: Huber, 1925. [German]

[2] Alexander F, French TM. Psychoanalytic therapy: Principles and application. New York: Ronald Press, 1946.

[3] Cordess C, Cox M, eds. Forensic psychotherapy. Crime, psychodynamics and the offender patient. (Vol. I and II). London: Jessica Kingsley, 1998.

[4] Welldon E, van Velsen C, eds. A practical guide to forensic psychotherapy. London: Jessica Kingsley, 1997.

[5] Eissler, R. The effect of the structure of the ego on psychoanalytic technique. J Am Psycho-analytic Assoc 1953;1:104-43.

[6] Fonagy P. Towards a developmental understanding of violence. Br J Psychiat 2003;183:190-2.

[7] Fonagy P. The developmental roots of violence in the failure of mentalization. In: Pfäfflin F, Adshead G, eds. A matter of security. The application of attachment theory to forensic psychiatry and psychotherapy. London: Jessica Kingsley, 2004:13-56.

[8] Hall GN. Sexual offender recidivism revisited: a meta-analysis of recent treatment studies. J Consult Clin Psychol 1995;63:802-9.

[9] Laws DR, Marshall WL. A brief history of behavioral and cognitive behavioral approaches to sexual offenders: Part 1. Early developments. Sex Abuse 2003;15:75-92.

[10] Marshall WL, Laws DR. A brief history of behavioral and cognitive behavioral approaches to sexual offender treatment: Part 2: The modern era. Sex Abuse 2003;15:93-120.

[11] Marshall WL, Fernandez Y, Hudson S, Ward T, eds. Sourcebook of treatment programs for sexual offenders. New York: Plenum Press, 1998.

[12] Hollin C, ed. The essential handbook of offender treatment and assessment. Chichester: John Wiley, 2004.

[13] Andrews D, Zinger I, Hoge RD, Bonta J, Gendreau P, Cullen FT. Does correctional treatment work? A clinically relevant and psychologically informed meta-analysis. Criminology 1990; 28:369-404.

[14] Andrews DA. Enhancing adherence to risk-need-responsivity. Crim Public Pol 2006;5:595-602.

[15] Andrews DA, Dowden C. Risk principle of case classification in correctional treatment: A meta-analytic investigation. Int J Offender Ther 2006;50:88-100.

[16] Miller WR, Rollnick S. Motivational Interviewing: preparing people for change, 2nd ed. New York: Guilford, 2002.

[17] Landenberger NA, Lipsey MW. The positive effects of cognitive-behavioral programs for offenders: A meta-analysis of factors associated with effective treatment. J Experimental Crim 2005;1:451-76.

[18] Lipsey MW. The evidence base for effective juvenile programs as a source for best practice guidelines. Nashville, TN: Vanderbilt Univ, Center Evaluat Res Methodol, 2006.

[19] Hanson RK, Bourgon G, Helmus L, Hodgson S. A meta-analysis of the effectiveness of treatment for sexual offenders: Risk, need, and responsivity. Corrections Research User Report No. 2009-01. Ottawa: Public Safety Canada, 2009.

[20] Lipsey MW, Cullen FT. The effectiveness of correctional rehabilitation: A review of systematic reviews. Annu Rev Law Soc Sci 2007; 3: 297-320.

[21] Lipsey MW. A standardized program evaluation protocol for programs serving juvenile probationers. Nashville, TN: Vanderbilt Univ, Center Evaluat Res Methodol, 2007.

[22] Howell JC. Preventing and reducing juvenile delinquency: A comprehensive framework, 2nd ed. Thousand Oaks, CA: Sage, 2009.

[23] Durlak JA, Lipsey MW. A practitioner´s guide to meta-analysis. Am J Community Psychol 1991;19:291-332.

[24] Ross RR, Fabiano EA, Ross RD. Reasoning and Rehabilitation: A handbook for teaching cognitive skills. Ottawa: Centre Cognit Dev, 1986.

[25] Goldstein AP, Sprafkin R, Gershaw NJ, Klein P. Skill streaming the adolescent. Champaign, IL: Res Press, 1980.

[26] Tong LSY, Farrington DP (2006). How effective is the "Reasoning and Rehabilitation" programme in reducing reoffending? A meta-analysis of evaluations in four countries. Psychol Crime Law 2006;12:3-24.

[27] Clarkin JF, Yeomans FE, Kernberg OF. Psychotherapy for Borderline Personality. New York: John Wiley, 1999.

[28] Clarkin JF, Levy KN, Lenzenweger MF, Kernberg OF. Evaluating three treatments for borderline personality disorder: A multiwave study. Am J Psychiat 2007;164:922-8.

[29] Bateman AW, Fonagy P. Mentalization-based treatment of BPD. J Pers Disord 2004;18:36-51.

[30] Yeomans FE, Clarkin JF, Kernberg OF (2002). A primer on transferencc-focused psychotherapy for the borderline patient. Northvale NJ: Jason Aronson, 2002.

[31] Mattke D, Dammann G, Martius P. Der Transfer von einzel-therapeutischen Behandlungskonzepten auf Gruppenformate: Das Beispiel der Übertragungsfokussierten Psychotherapie (TFP) [The transfer of individual treatment concepts on group settings. The example of Transference Focused Psychotherapy (TFP)]. Gruppenpsychother GR 2007; 43: 161-80. [German]

[32] Fontao MI, Pfäfflin F, Lamott F. Anwendung der TFP auf die Behandlung von Maßregelvollzugspatienten. Eine Pilotstudie. [Application of TFP in the treatment of forensic psychiatric patients - a pilot study] In: Lackinger F, Dammann G, Wittmann B, eds. Psychodynamische Psychotherapie bei Delinquenz. Stuttgart: Schattauer, 2008: 395-405. [German]

[33] Fonagy P, Bateman AW. Mechanisms of change in mentalization-based treatment of BPD. J Clin Psychol 2006;62:411-30.

[34] Bateman AW, Fonagy P. 8-Year follow-up of patients reated for borderline personality disorder: Mentalization-based treatment versus treatment as usual. Am J Psychiat 2008;165:631-8.

[35] Twemlow SW, Fonagy P, Sacco FC. An innovative psychodynamically influenced approach to reduce school violence. J Am Acad Child Psy 2001;40:377-9.

[36] Twemlow SW, Fonagy P, Sacco FC. The role of the bystander in the social architecture of bullying and violence in schools and communities. In: Devine J, Gilligan J, Miczek KA, Shaikh R, Pfaff D, eds. Youth violence: scientific approaches to prevention. New York: NY Acad Sci, 2004:215-32.

[37] Twemlow SW, Fonagy P. Transforming violent social systems into non-violent mentalizing systems: an experiment in schools. In: Allen JG, Fonagy P, eds. The handbook of mentalization-based treatment. Hoboken: John Wiley, 2006:289-306.

[38] Bateman AW, Fonagy P. Comorbid antisocial and borderline personality disorders: mentalization-based treatment. J Clin Psychol 2008;64: 181-94.

[39] McGuire J. Criminal sanctions versus psychologically based interventions with offenders: a comparative empirical analysis. Psychol Crime Law 2002;8:183-208.
[40] Marshall WL, McGuire J. Effect sizes in the treatment of sexual offenders. Int J Offender Ther 2003;47:653-663.
[41] Lipsey MW. The effect of treatment on juvenile delinquents: Results from meta-analysis. In: Lösel F, Bender D, Bliesener T, eds. Psychology and Law. International Perspectives. Berlin: De Gruyter, 1992:131-43.
[42] Lipsey MW, Wilson DB. The efficacy of psychological educational and behavioural treatment. Am Psychol 1993;48:1181-1209.
[43] Lösel F. The efficacy of correctional treatment: A review and synthesis of meta-evaluations. In: McGuire J, ed. What works: Reducing re-offending: Guidelines from research and practice. Chichester: John Wiley, 1995: 79-111.
[44] Redondo S, Sanchez-Meca J, Garrido V. The influence of treatment programmes on the recidivism of juvenile and adult offenders: A European meta-analytic review. Psychol Crime Law 1999;5:251-78.
[45] Egg R, Pearson FS, Cleland CM, Lipton DS. Evaluation von Straftäterbehandlungsprogrammen in Deutschland: Überblick und Meta-Analyse. [Evaluation of offender treatment programmes in Germany: An overview and meta-analysis]. In: Rehn G, Wischka B, Lösel F, Walter M, eds. Behandlung gefährlicher Straftäter. Grundlagen Konzepte Ergebnisse. Herbolzheim: Centaurus, 2001:321-47 [German]
[46] Hanson RK, Gordon A, Harris AJ, Marques JK, Murphy W, Quinsey VL, Seto MC. First report of the collaborative outcome data project on the effectiveness of psychological treatment for sex offenders. Sex Abuse 2002;14:169-94.
[47] Lambert M, ed. Bergin and Garfield's Handbook of psychotherapy and behavior change. New York: John Wiley, 2004.
[48] Welsh BC, Farrington DP. Correctional intervention programs and cost benefit analysis. Crim Justice Behav 2000;27:115-33.
[49] Pearson FS, Lipton DS, Cleland CM, Yee DS. The effects of behavioural/cognitive behavioural programs on recidivism. Crime Delinquency 2002;48:476-96.
[50] Dowden C, Antonowicz D, Andrews DA. The effectiveness of relapse prevention with offenders: a meta-analysis. Int J Offender Ther 2003;47: 516-28.
[51] Walker DF, McGovern SK, Poey EL, Otis KE. Treatment effectiveness for male adolescent sexual offenders: a meta-analysis and review. J Child Sex Abuse 2004;13:281-93.
[52] Lösel F, Schmucker M. The effectiveness of treatment for sexual offenders: A comprehensive meta-analysis. J Experimental Crim 2005;1: 117-46.
[53] Sherman LW, Farrington DP, MacKenzie DL, Welsh BC. Evidence based crime prevention. New York: Routledge, 2006.
[54] Reitzel LR, Carbonell JL. The effectiveness of sexual offender treatment for juveniles as measured by recidivism: A meta-analysis. Sex Abuse 2006;18:401-21.
[55] Ward T, Brown M. The Good Lives Model and conceptual issues in offender rehabilitation. Psychol Crime Law 2004;10:243-57.
[56] Ward T, Gannon TA. Rehabilitation etiology and self-regulation: the comprehensive good lives model of treatment for sexual offenders. Aggress Violent Behav 2006;11:77-94.
[57] Ross T. Current issues in self regulation research and their significance for therapeutic intervention in offender groups. Int J Behav Consultation Ther 2008;4:68-81.
[58] Farrington DP (2003). Key results from the first 40 years of the Cambridge Study in Delinquent Development. In: Thornberry TP, Krohn MD, eds. Taking stock of Delinquency: an overview of findings from contemporary longitudinal studies. New York: Kluwer/Plenum, 2003: 137-84.
[59] Loeber R, Farrington DP, eds. Serious and violent juvenile offenders: Risk factors and successful interventions. Thousand Oaks, CA: Sage, 1998.
[60] Loeber R, Farrington DP, eds. Child delinquents. Development Intervention and service needs. Thousand Oaks CA: Sage, 2001.
[61] Loeber R, Farrington DP, Stouthamer-Loeber M, White HR. Violence and serious theft: Development and prediction from childhood to adulthood. New York: Routledge, 2008.

[62] Durlak JA. Common risk and protective factors in successful prevention programs. Am J Orthopsychiat 1998;68:512-20.

SECTION THREE: ACKNOWLEDGEMENTS

In: School, Adolescence and Health Issues
Editors: J. Merrick, A. Tenenbaum and H. A. Omar
ISBN: 978-1-62948-702-1

Chapter 18

ABOUT THE EDITORS

Joav Merrick, MD, MMedSci, DMSc, born in Copenhagen, is professor of pediatrics, child health and human development affiliated with Kentucky Children's Hospital, University of Kentucky, Lexington, Kentucky, United States and the Division of Pediatrics, Hadassah Hebrew University Medical Center, Mt Scopus Campus, Jerusalem, Israel, the medical director of the Health Services, Division for Intellectual and Developmental Disabilities, Ministry of Social Affairs and Social Services, Jerusalem, the founder and director of the National Institute of Child Health and Human Development in Israel. Numerous publications in the field of pediatrics, child health and human development, rehabilitation, intellectual disability, disability, health, welfare, abuse, advocacy, quality of life and prevention. Received the Peter Sabroe Child Award for outstanding work on behalf of Danish Children in 1985 and the International LEGO-Prize ("The Children's Nobel Prize") for an extraordinary contribution towards improvement in child welfare and well-being in 1987. E-mail: jmerrick@zahav.net.il

Ariel Tenenbaum, MD, born in Argentina, graduated from the Hadassah Hebrew University Medical School in Jerusalem, Israel. Specialist in pediatrics and the director of the Down Syndrome Center and the Intellectual and Developmental Disability Evaluation Center at the Department of Pediatrics, Hadassah Hebrew University Medical Centers, Mt Scopus Campus, Jerusalem. Medical consultant at the Feeding Disorder Clinic, and director of the Pre-adoption Evaluation Clinic. Several publications in the field of pediatric medicine, child and public health and especially around medical conditions in persons with Down syndrome. E-mail: tene@hadassah.org.il

Hatim A Omar, MD, FAAP, Professor of Pediatrics and Obstetrics and Gynecology; Professor of Family Studies; and Chief of the Division of Adolescent Medicine, Department of Pediatrics, University of Kentucky, Lexington. He is the holder of the Children's Miracle Network Endowed Chair in Pediatrics. Dr. Omar has completed residency training in obstetrics and gynecology as well as pediatrics. He has also completed fellowships in vascular physiology and adolescent medicine. He is the recipient of the Commonwealth of Kentucky Governor's Award for community service and volunteerism in 2000, Kentucky Teen Pregnancy Coalition Award for outstanding service 2002, Awards for suicide prevention from the Ohio Valley Society for Adolescent Medicine and Kentucky Pediatric Society in 2005 and

2007, Sexual Abuse Awareness Month Award for his work with sexual abuse victims from the Kentucky Association of Sexual Assault Professionals in 2007, Special Achievement Award from the American Academy of Pediatrics 2007 and the Founders of Adolescent Medicine Award from the AAP in 2007. He is well known internationally with numerous publications in child health, public health, pediatrics, adolescent medicine, pediatric and adolescent gynecology. E-mail: haomar2@uky.edu

In: School, Adolescence and Health Issues
Editors: J. Merrick, A. Tenenbaum and H. A. Omar
ISBN: 978-1-62948-702-1

Chapter 19

About the National Institute of Child Health and Human Development in Israel

The National Institute of Child Health and Human Development (NICHD) in Israel was established in 1998 as a virtual institute under the auspicies of the Medical Director, Ministry of Social Affairs and Social Services in order to function as the research arm for the Office of the Medical Director. In 1998 the National Council for Child Health and Pediatrics, Ministry of Health and in 1999 the Director General and Deputy Director General of the Ministry of Health endorsed the establishment of the NICHD.

Mission

The mission of a National Institute for Child Health and Human Development in Israel is to provide an academic focal point for the scholarly interdisciplinary study of child life, health, public health, welfare, disability, rehabilitation, intellectual disability and related aspects of human development. This mission includes research, teaching, clinical work, information and public service activities in the field of child health and human development.

Service and academic activities

Over the years many activities became focused in the south of Israel due to collaboration with various professionals at the Faculty of Health Sciences (FOHS) at the Ben Gurion University of the Negev (BGU). Since 2000 an affiliation with the Zusman Child Development Center at the Pediatric Division of Soroka University Medical Center has resulted in collaboration around the establishment of the Down Syndrome Clinic at that center. In 2002 a full course on "Disability" was established at the Recanati School for Allied Professions in the Community, FOHS, BGU and in 2005 collaboration was started with the Primary Care Unit of the faculty and disability became part of the master of public health course on "Children and society". In the academic year 2005-2006 a one semester course on "Aging with disability" was started as part of the master of science program in gerontology in our collaboration with the Center for Multidisciplinary Research in Aging. In 2010 collaborations with the Division of Pediatrics, Hadassah Hebrew University Medical Center, Jerusalem, Israel around the National Down Syndrome Center and teaching students and residents about intellectual and developmental disabilities as part of their training at this campus.

Research activities

The affiliated staff have over the years published work from projects and research activities in this national and international collaboration. In the year 2000 the International Journal of Adolescent Medicine and Health and in 2005 the International Journal on Disability and Human Development of De Gruyter Publishing House (Berlin and New York) were affiliated with the National Institute of Child Health and Human Development. From 2008 also the International Journal of Child Health and Human Development (Nova Science, New York), the International Journal of Child and Adolescent Health (Nova Science) and the Journal of Pain Management (Nova Science) affiliated and from 2009 the International Public Health Journal (Nova Science) and Journal of Alternative Medicine Research (Nova Science). All peer-reviewed international journals.

National collaborations

Nationally the NICHD works in collaboration with the Faculty of Health Sciences, Ben Gurion University of the Negev; Department of Physical Therapy, Sackler School of Medicine, Tel Aviv University; Autism Center, Assaf HaRofeh Medical Center; National Rett and PKU Centers at Chaim Sheba Medical Center, Tel HaShomer; Department of Physiotherapy, Haifa University; Department of Education, Bar Ilan University, Ramat Gan, Faculty of Social Sciences and Health Sciences; College of Judea and Samaria in Ariel and in 2011 affiliation with Center for Pediatric Chronic Diseases and National Center for Down Syndrome, Department of Pediatrics, Hadassah Hebrew University Medical Center, Mount Scopus Campus, Jerusalem.

International collaborations

Internationally with the Department of Disability and Human Development, College of Applied Health Sciences, University of Illinois at Chicago; Strong Center for Developmental Disabilities, Golisano Children's Hospital at Strong, University of Rochester School of Medicine and Dentistry, New York; Centre on Intellectual Disabilities, University of Albany, New York; Centre for Chronic Disease Prevention and Control, Health Canada, Ottawa; Chandler Medical Center and Children's Hospital, Kentucky Children's Hospital, Section of Adolescent Medicine, University of Kentucky, Lexington; Chronic Disease Prevention and Control Research Center, Baylor College of Medicine, Houston, Texas; Division of Neuroscience, Department of Psychiatry, Columbia University, New York; Institute for the Study of Disadvantage and Disability, Atlanta; Center for Autism and Related Disorders, Department Psychiatry, Children's Hospital Boston, Boston; Department of Paediatrics, Child Health and Adolescent Medicine, Children's Hospital at Westmead, Westmead,

Australia; International Centre for the Study of Occupational and Mental Health, Düsseldorf, Germany; Centre for Advanced Studies in Nursing, Department of General Practice and Primary Care, University of Aberdeen, Aberdeen, United Kingdom; Quality of Life Research Center, Copenhagen, Denmark; Nordic School of Public Health, Gottenburg, Sweden, Scandinavian Institute of Quality of Working Life, Oslo, Norway; The Department of Applied Social Sciences (APSS) of The Hong Kong Polytechnic University Hong Kong.

Targets

Our focus is on research, international collaborations, clinical work, teaching and policy in health, disability and human development and to establish the NICHD as a permanent institute at one of the residential care centers for persons with intellectual disability in Israel in order to conduct model research and together with the four university schools of public health/medicine in Israel establish a national master and doctoral program in disability and human development at the institute to secure the next generation of professionals working in this often non-prestigious/low-status field of work.

Contact

Joav Merrick, MD, MMedSci, DMSc
Professor of Pediatrics, Child Health and Human Development
Medical Director, Health Services, Division for Intellectual and Developmental Disabilities, Ministry of Social Affairs and Social Services, POB 1260, IL-91012 Jerusalem, Israel.
E-mail: jmerrick@zahav.net.il

In: School, Adolescence and Health Issues
Editors: J. Merrick, A. Tenenbaum and H. A. Omar
ISBN: 978-1-62948-702-1

Chapter 20

About the Division of Adolescent Medicine, Kentucky Children's Hospital at the University of Kentucky, Lexington, Kentucky, United States

The Kentucky Children's Hospital is the only facility in central and eastern Kentucky dedicated to the expert medical and surgical care of infants, children and adolescents. The University of Kentucky (UK) has a proud and distinguished history of providing comprehensive programs and innovative care to the children of the region. Although patients are referred from every county of the Commonwealth of Kentucky and from every adjacent state, the majority of patients are from the Bluegrass region around Lexington and from Appalachian counties in the eastern part of Kentucky. The Department of Pediatrics has provided service and education from the opening of UK College of Medicine in 1961.

The passion for teaching is palpable at the Kentucky Children's Hospital. Most years about 15% of our graduates or more choose to train in pediatrics. The University of Kentucky had one of the earliest combined Internal Medicine-Pediatrics residency program with "med-peds" graduates very well represented throughout the faculty. This, in addition to a strong adolescent medicine program, is among factors which have led to a focus upon adolescent and adult graduates of pediatric care from Kentucky Children's Hospital.

The approach at the Kentucky Children's Hospital (KCH) is focused on family-centered care. Full-time child life coverage, facilities for families to stay with children overnight, age-appropriate playrooms, children's library facilities, in-hospital school services, a dedicated television channel, a computer laboratory and many other features provide the special environment to provide the best of care for children. The Kentucky Children's Hospital includes a 12-bed Pediatric Intensive Care Unit, a 66 bed Level 3 Neonatal Intensive Care Unit, 44 acute care pediatric beds, a 26 bed normal newborn nursery, and an 8 bed short stay admissions/observation unit. KCH has grown from about 3,750 discharges per year in 2004 to about 5,400 in 2009.

Pediatric medical and surgical outpatient facilities are primarily located in the Kentucky Clinic, which is attached to the hospital. Each year, the pediatric clinic has over 46,000 patient visits. Of these, over 15,300 patient visits are in the general pediatric and continuity clinics, over 17,400 occur in the various subspecialty clinics. Kentucky Children's Twilight

Clinic is open all but two days of the year in addition to the state-of –the-art pediatric emergency center.

Specialty care includes medical and surgical cardiac care, endocrinology, pediatric kidney disease, developmental pediatrics, pediatric allergy and immunology, solid organ transplantation, behavioral pediatrics, pediatric emergency medicine, intensive care pediatrics, neonatology, gastroenterology and hepatology, dysmorphology, biochemical genetics, pediatric rheumatology, oncology, hematology, infectious diseases, hospitalist care, adolescent medicine, adolescent gynecology, child neurology, pediatric surgery, pediatric orthopedics, pediatric imaging, child psychiatry, pediatric anesthesiology, pediatric otorhinolaryngology, speech disorders, pediatric pathology, pediatric physical medicine, pediatric neurosurgery and many other fields. The Young Parents Program is an innovative service of the Adolescent Medicine Division, which has been very successful. Many of these specialties cover outreach clinics throughout underserved Appalachian counties of Kentucky as well as in Lexington. New facilities are in preparation, because of the remarkable growth in clinical programs for children.

The growth of clinical programs and service capability has been matched by considerable growth in pediatric research at UK. Substantial programs in vascular biology and diabetes, pediatric inflammatory biology, molecular pediatrics, developmental biology, pediatric health policy research, epidemiology, prevention, cancer research and pediatric pharmacology are growing rapidly. The Kentucky Children's Hospital is located on the UK campus. Access to faculty in the other colleges including social sciences and humanities enhances the Kentucky Children's Hospital scholarly environment and provides unique opportunities for collaborative work.

As we approach our 50th year anniversary, we remain committed to improving the lives and health of young people of the Commonwealth and improving the future for their families.

Division of Adolescent Medicine

The Division of Adolescent Medicine was founded in 1998 to provide state of the art care for adolescent patients from all areas of the commonwealth of Kentucky, to serve as a state wide resource for education and training for local providers on adolescent issues, to study specific factors on the local level affecting youth in the state, to help teach medical students and residents and to provide community service to help improve teen future in the commonwealth.

The division provides comprehensive, holistic team approach to adolescents, where teens receive all aspects of care from mental health to routine care from a team of professionals including physicians, mental health providers, social workers, psychologists, nutritionists and nursing staff. One unique program within the division is the Young Parent Program, where pregnant teens are cared for throughout pregnancy then they and their babies are cared for together in the program.

The division is active in research with many peer reviewed articles published each year as well as several books and special journal editions.

In the community, the program has founded several grass route programs to help prevent youth suicide, teen pregnancy, accidental death and substance abuse among adolescents in Kentucky.

The division has provided more than 300 lectures, workshops, media events and teaching for community providers, parents, teachers and school counselors. It also provides advocacy work on behalf of teens with active work at the state legislative and executive government as well as local governments to help improve the lives of teens.

Collaborations

The Division of Adolescent Medicine collaborates locally with school boards, youth service centers, state and local governments, other universities and child advocacy centers as well as with regional adolescent medicine programs.

Internationally with the Institute for Child Health and Human Development in Israel, the Division of Adolescent Medicine at Santa Casa University, Brazil, Quality of Life Research Center and Nordic School of Holistic Health, Copenhagen, Denmark, Department of Applied Social Sciences, The Hong Kong Polytechnic University, Hong Kong.

The vision

The vision of the Division of Adolescent Medicine is to improve the health and long term wellbeing of Kentucky Youth to grow into productive adults. We also invision global work to help positive youth development world wide.

Target areas of interests

The interest areas of the division are all aspects of youth development and adolescent health with focus on prevention and community involvement in collaboration on the local, national and global level with programs having the same goal.

Contact

Hatim Omar, MD, FAAP
Professor of Pediatrics and Obstetrics/Gynecology
Director of Adolescent Medicine & Young Parent programs
J422, Kentucky Clinic
Department of Pediatrics, Kentucky Children's Hospital
University of Kentucky College of Medicine
Lexington, KY 40536
E-mail: haomar2@uky.edu
Website://www.mc.uky.edu/

In: School, Adolescence and Health Issues
Editors: J. Merrick, A. Tenenbaum and H. A. Omar
ISBN: 978-1-62948-702-1

Chapter 21

About the Book Series "Pediatrics, Child and Adolescent Health"

Pediatrics, child and adolescent health is a book series with publications from a multidisciplinary group of researchers, practitioners and clinicians for an international professional forum interested in the broad spectrum of pediatric medicine, child health, adolescent health and human development.

- Merrick J, ed. Child and adolescent health yearbook 2011. New York: Nova Science, 2012.
- Merrick J, ed. Child and adolescent health yearbook 2012. New York: Nova Science, 2012.
- Roach RR, Greydanus DE, Patel DR, Homnick DN, Merrick J, eds. Tropical pediatrics: A public health concern of international proportions. New York: Nova Science, 2012.
- Merrick J, ed. Child health and human development yearbook 2011. New York: Nova Science, 2012.
- Merrick J, ed. Child health and human development yearbook 2012. New York: Nova Science, 2012.
- Shek DTL, Sun RCF, Merrick J, eds. Developmental issues in Chinese adolescents. New York: Nova Science, 2012.
- Shek DTL, Sun RCF, Merrick J, eds. Positive youth development: Theory, research and application. New York: Nova Science, 2012.
- Zachor DA, Merrick J, eds. Understanding autism spectrum disorder: Current research aspects. New York: Nova Science, 2012.
- Ma HK, Shek DTL, Merrick J, eds. Positive youth development: A new school curriculum to tackle adolescent developmental issues. New York: Nova Science, 2012.
- Wood D, Reiss JG, Ferris ME, Edwards LR, Merrick J, eds. Transition from pediatric to adult medical care. New York: Nova Science, 2012.
- Isenberg Y. Guidelines for the healthy integration of the ill child in the educational system: Experience from Israel. New York: Nova Science, 2013.
- Shek DTL, Sun RCF, Merrick J, eds. Chinese adolescent development: Economic disadvantages, parents and intrapersonal development. New York: Nova Science, 2013.

- Shek DTL, Sun RCF, Merrick J, eds. University and college students: Health and development issues for the leaders of tomorrow. New York: Nova Science, 2013.
- Shek DTL, Sun RCF, Merrick J, eds. Adolescence and behavior issues in a Chinese context. New York: Nova Science, 2013.
- Sun J, Buys N, Merrick J. Advances in preterm infant research. New York: Nova Science, 2013.
- Tsitsika A, Janikian M, Greydanus DE, Omar HA, Merrick J, eds. Internet addiction: A public health concern in adolescence. New York: Nova Science, 2013.
- Shek, DTL, Lee TY, Merrick J, eds. Promotion of holistic development of young people in Hong Kong. New York: Nova Science, 2013.
- Shek DTL, Ma C, Lu Y, Merrick J, eds. Human developmental research: Experience from research in Hong Kong. New York: Nova Science, 2013.
- Merrick J, ed. Chronic disease and disability in childhood. New York: Nova Science, 2013.
- Rubin IL, Merrick J, eds. Break the cycle of environmental health disparities: Maternal and child health aspects. New York: Nova Science, 2013.
- Rubin IL, Merrick J, eds. Environmental health disparities in children: Asthma, obesity and food. New York: Nova Science, 2013.
- Rubin IL, Merrick J, eds. Environmental health: Home, school and community. New York: Nova Science, 2013.
- Rubin IL, Merrick J, eds. Child health and human development: Social, economic and environmental factors. New York: Nova Science, 2013.

Contact

Professor Joav Merrick, MD, MMedSci, DMSc
Medical Director, Medical Services
Division for Intellectual and Developmental Disabilities
Ministry of Social Affairs and Social Services
POBox 1260, IL-91012 Jerusalem, Israel
E-mail: jmerrick@zahav.net.il

SECTION FOUR: INDEX

INDEX

A

D

I

J

K

L

M

N

O

P

Q

R

S